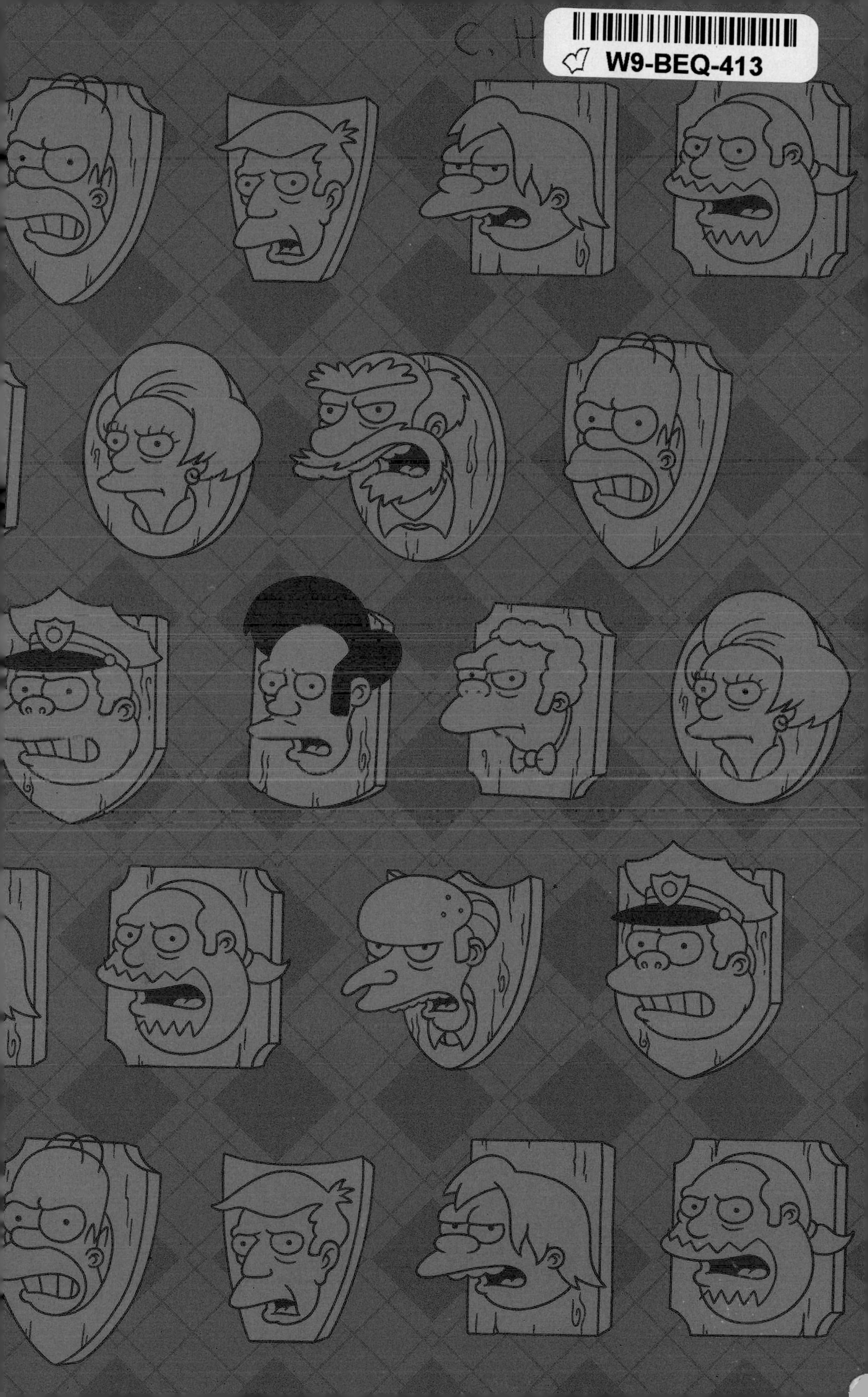

BIG BEASTLY BOOK OF
BART SIMPSON

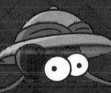

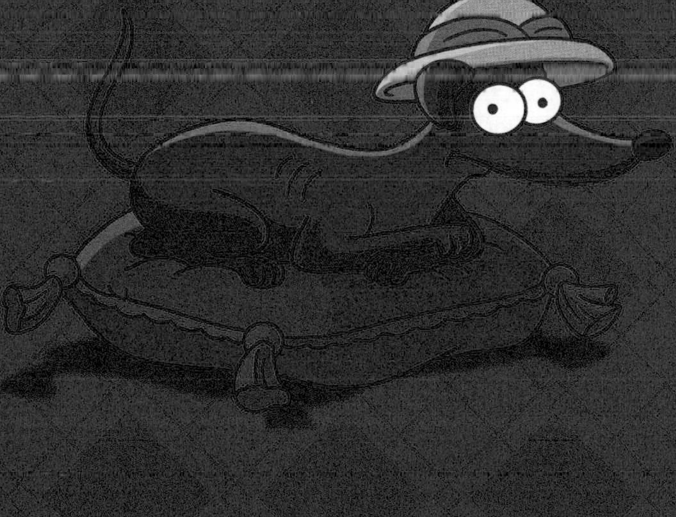

HARPER

NEW YORK • LONDON • TORONTO • SYDNEY

BIG BEASTLY BOOK OF BART SIMPSON

HarperCollins books may be purchased for educational, business, or sales
promotional use. For information please write
Special Markets Department,
HarperCollins Publishers,
10 East 53rd Street, New York, NY 10022.

FIRST EDITION

ISBN: 978-0-06-123128-5
ISBN-10: 0-06-123128-2

07 08 09 00 11 QWM 10 9 8 7 6 5 4 3 2 1

Publisher: MATT GROENING
Creative Director: BILL MORRISON
Managing Editor: TERRY DELEGEANE
Director of Operations: ROBERT ZAUGH
Art Director: NATHAN KANE
Art Director Special Projects: SERBAN CRISTESCU
Production Manager: CHRISTOPHER UNGAR
Legal Guardian: SUSAN A. GRODE
HarperCollins Editors: HOPE INNELLI, JEREMY CESAREC

Trade Paperback Concepts and Design: SERBAN CRISTESCU

Contributing Artists:
KAREN BATES, JOHN COSTANZA, SERBAN CRISTESCU, JOHN DELANEY,
LUIS ESCOBAR, NATHAN HAMILL, JASON HO, NATHAN KANE, JAMES LLOYD,
JEANETTE MORENO, BILL MORRISON, PHYLLIS NOVIN, PHIL ORTIZ, PATRICK OWSLEY,
ANDREW PEPOY, MIKE ROTE, HOWARD SHUM, ART VILLANUEVA, CHRIS UNGAR

Contributing Writers:
JAMES W. BATES, TONY DIGEROLAMO, TOM PEYER, ERIC ROGERS

PRINTED IN CANADA

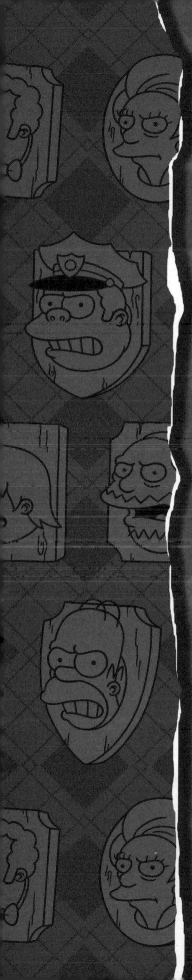

TABLE OF CONTENTS

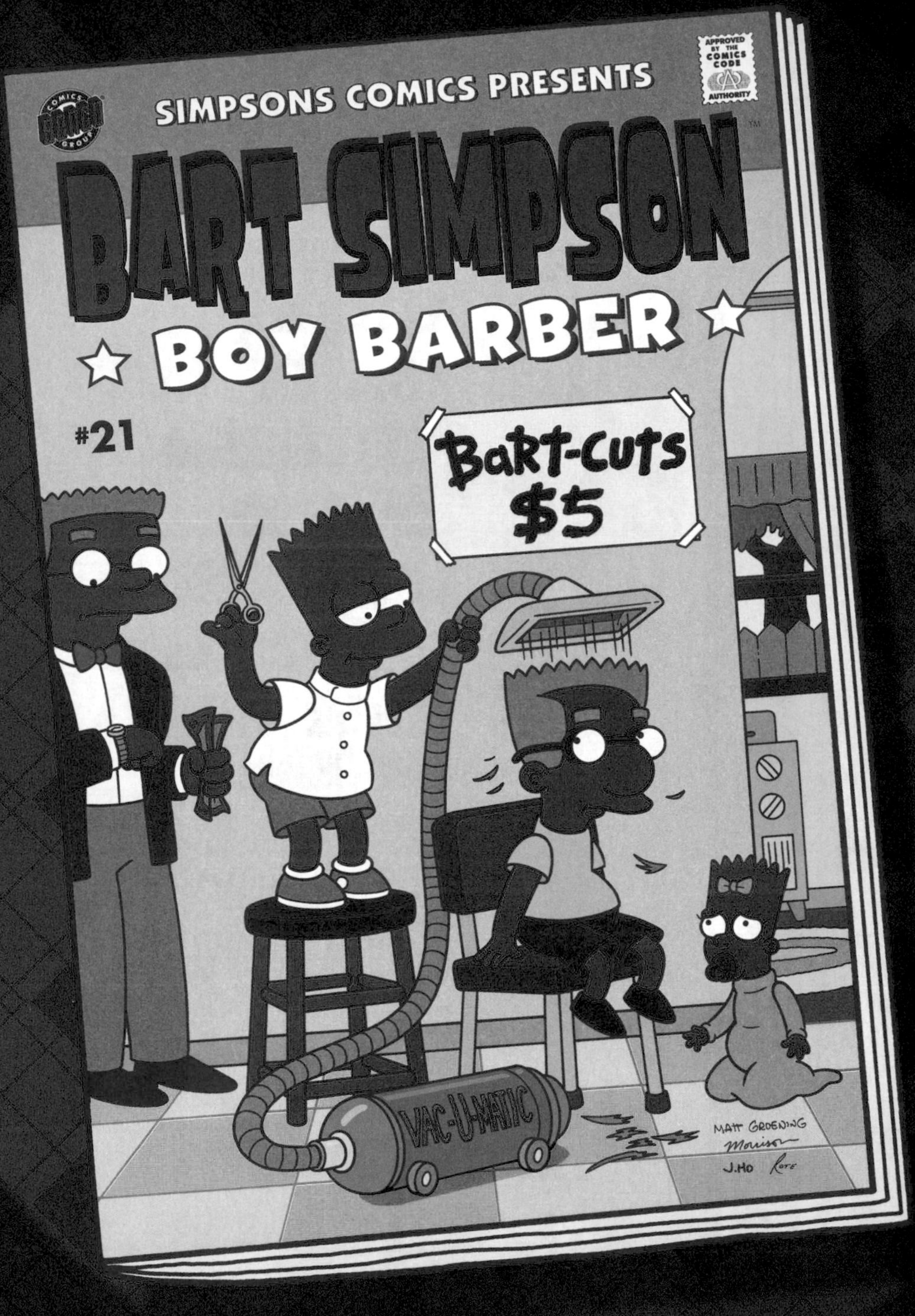
APPROVED BY THE COMICS CODE AUTHORITY
SIMPSONS COMICS PRESENTS
BART SIMPSON
BOY BARBER
#21
BART-CUTS
$5
VAC-U-MATIC
MATT GROENING
J.HO

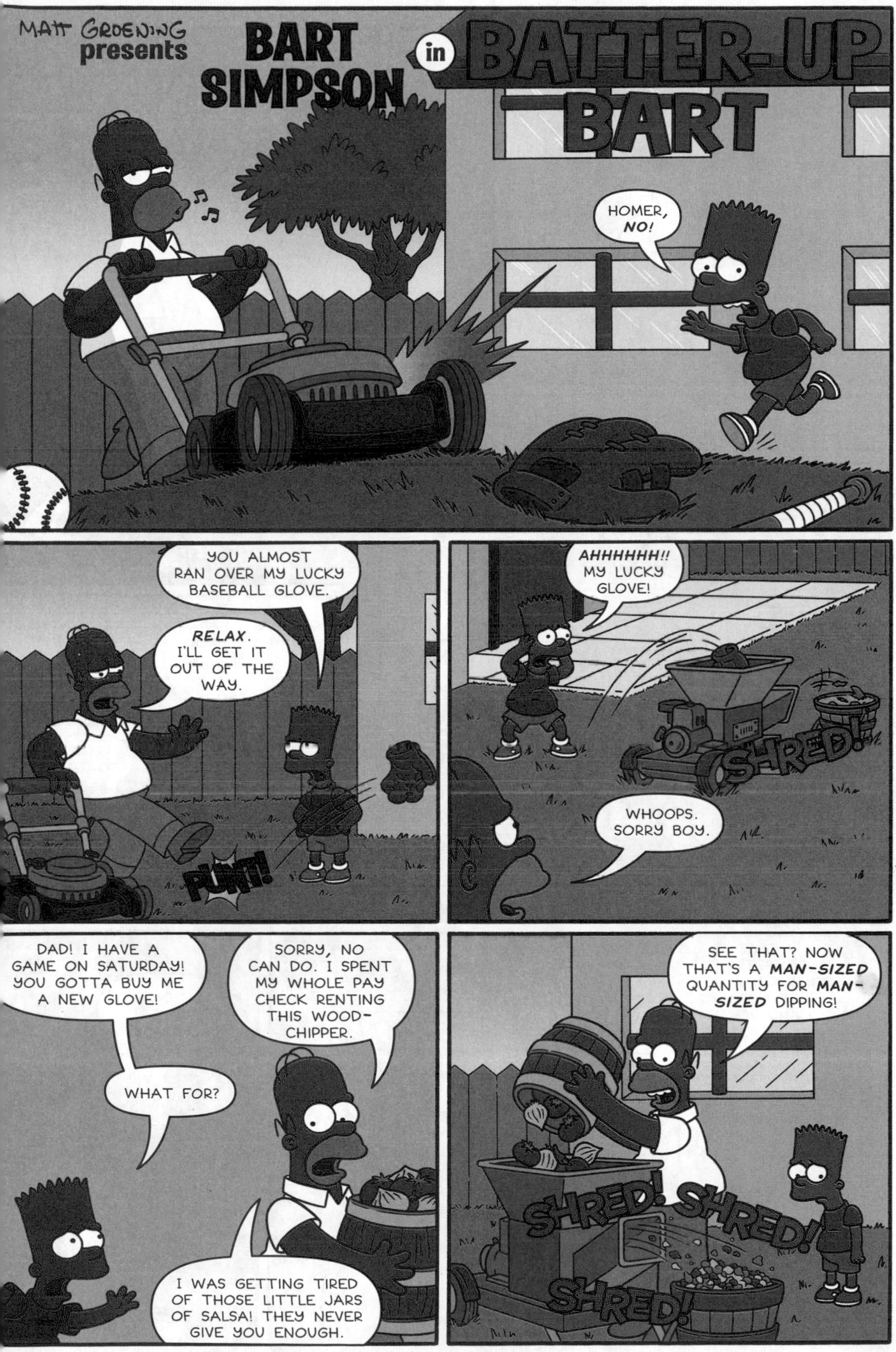
MATT GROENING presents
BART SIMPSON in BATTER-UP BART
HOMER, NO!
YOU ALMOST RAN OVER MY LUCKY BASEBALL GLOVE.
RELAX. I'LL GET IT OUT OF THE WAY.
PUNT!
AHHHHHH!! MY LUCKY GLOVE!
SHRED!
WHOOPS. SORRY BOY.
DAD! I HAVE A GAME ON SATURDAY! YOU GOTTA BUY ME A NEW GLOVE!
SORRY, NO CAN DO. I SPENT MY WHOLE PAY CHECK RENTING THIS WOOD-CHIPPER.
WHAT FOR?
I WAS GETTING TIRED OF THOSE LITTLE JARS OF SALSA! THEY NEVER GIVE YOU ENOUGH.
SEE THAT? NOW THAT'S A MAN-SIZED QUANTITY FOR MAN-SIZED DIPPING!
SHRED! SHRED!
SHRED!

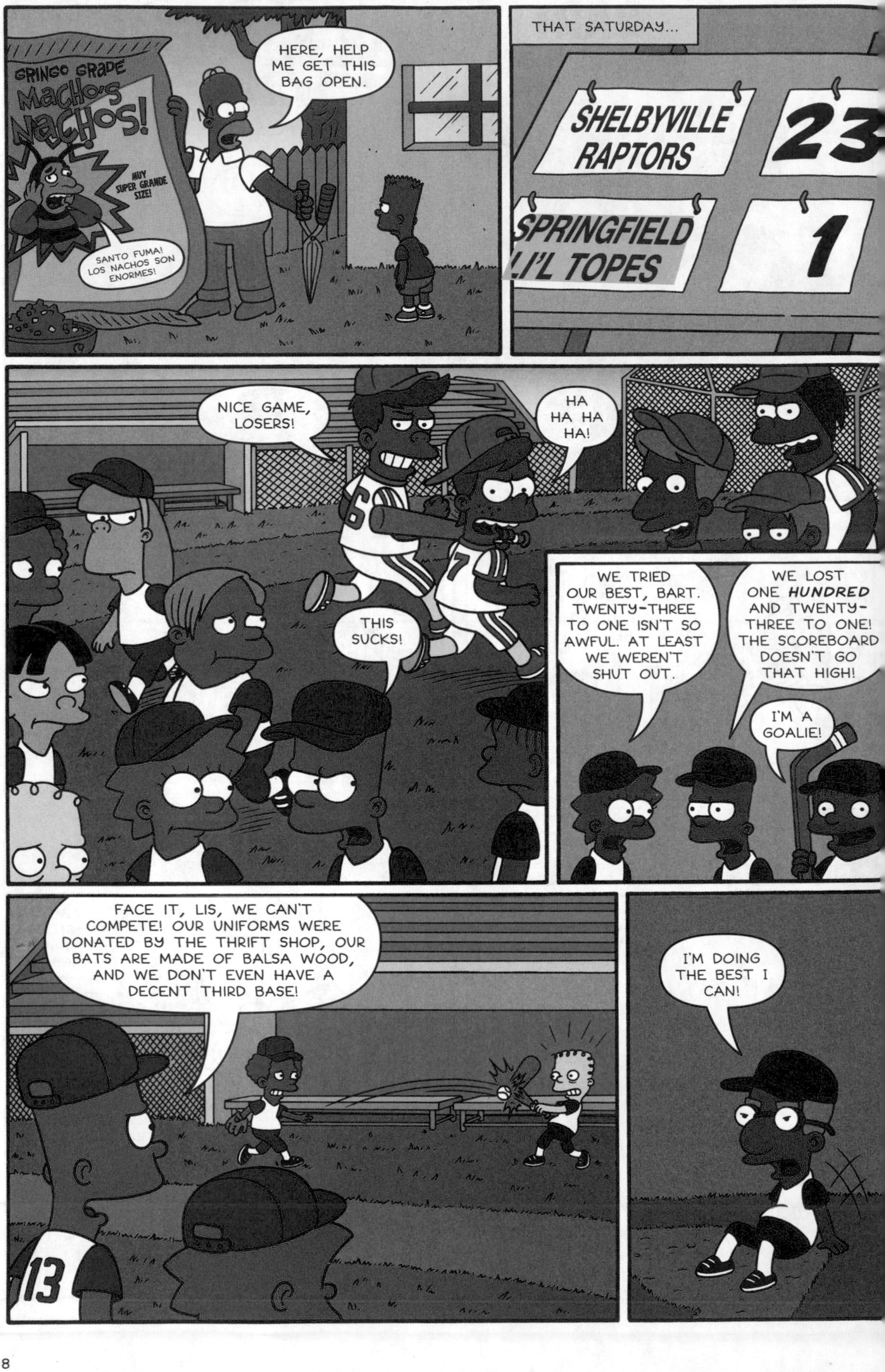
GRINGO GRADE
MACHO'S NACHOS!
MUY SUPER GRANDE SIZE!
SANTO FUMA! LOS NACHOS SON ENORMES!
HERE, HELP ME GET THIS BAG OPEN.
THAT SATURDAY...
SHELBYVILLE RAPTORS
23
SPRINGFIELD LI'L TOPES
1
NICE GAME, LOSERS!
HA HA HA HA!
THIS SUCKS!
WE TRIED OUR BEST, BART. TWENTY-THREE TO ONE ISN'T SO AWFUL. AT LEAST WE WEREN'T SHUT OUT.
WE LOST ONE HUNDRED AND TWENTY-THREE TO ONE! THE SCOREBOARD DOESN'T GO THAT HIGH!
I'M A GOALIE!
FACE IT, LIS, WE CAN'T COMPETE! OUR UNIFORMS WERE DONATED BY THE THRIFT SHOP, OUR BATS ARE MADE OF BALSA WOOD, AND WE DON'T EVEN HAVE A DECENT THIRD BASE!
I'M DOING THE BEST I CAN!

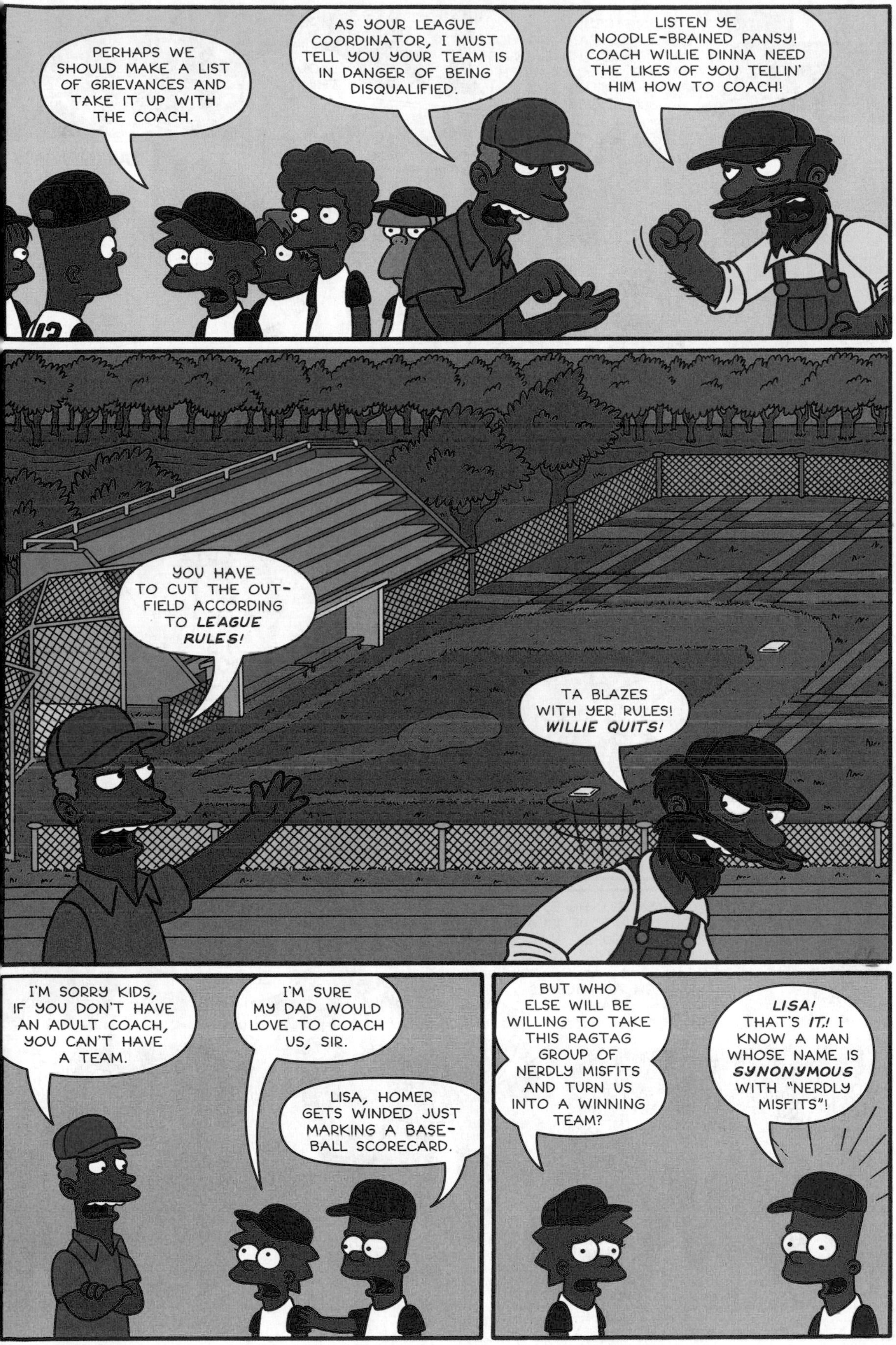
PERHAPS WE SHOULD MAKE A LIST OF GRIEVANCES AND TAKE IT UP WITH THE COACH.
AS YOUR LEAGUE COORDINATOR, I MUST TELL YOU YOUR TEAM IS IN DANGER OF BEING DISQUALIFIED.
LISTEN YE NOODLE-BRAINED PANSY! COACH WILLIE DINNA NEED THE LIKES OF YOU TELLIN' HIM HOW TO COACH!
YOU HAVE TO CUT THE OUT-FIELD ACCORDING TO LEAGUE RULES!
TA BLAZES WITH YER RULES! WILLIE QUITS!
I'M SORRY KIDS, IF YOU DON'T HAVE AN ADULT COACH, YOU CAN'T HAVE A TEAM.
I'M SURE MY DAD WOULD LOVE TO COACH US, SIR.
LISA, HOMER GETS WINDED JUST MARKING A BASE-BALL SCORECARD.
BUT WHO ELSE WILL BE WILLING TO TAKE THIS RAGTAG GROUP OF NERDLY MISFITS AND TURN US INTO A WINNING TEAM?
LISA! THAT'S IT! I KNOW A MAN WHOSE NAME IS SYNONYMOUS WITH "NERDLY MISFITS"!

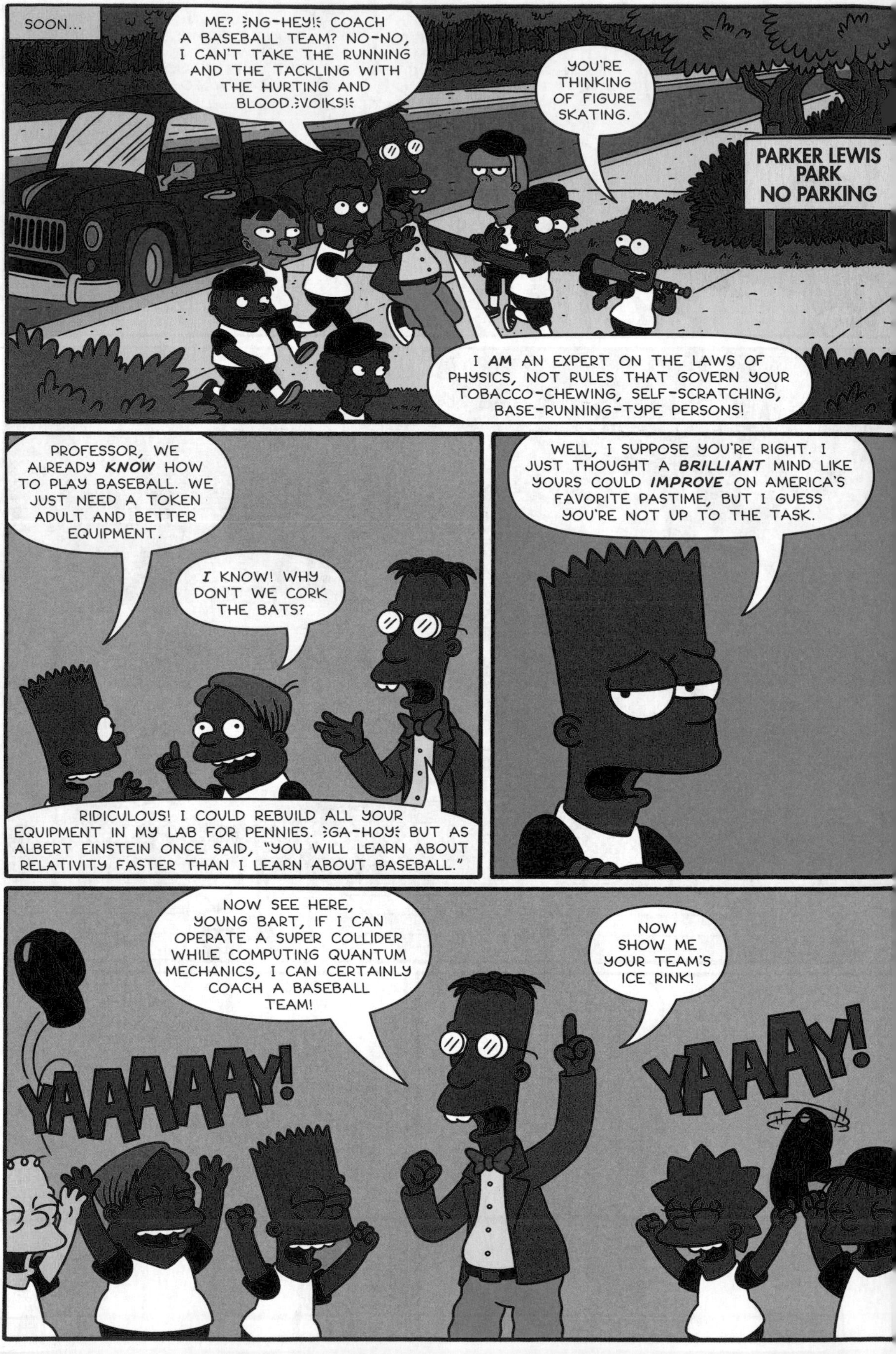
SOON...
ME? ⁝NG-HEY!⁝ COACH A BASEBALL TEAM? NO-NO, I CAN'T TAKE THE RUNNING AND THE TACKLING WITH THE HURTING AND BLOOD.⁝VOIKS!⁝
YOU'RE THINKING OF FIGURE SKATING.
PARKER LEWIS PARK NO PARKING
I AM AN EXPERT ON THE LAWS OF PHYSICS, NOT RULES THAT GOVERN YOUR TOBACCO-CHEWING, SELF-SCRATCHING, BASE-RUNNING-TYPE PERSONS!
PROFESSOR, WE ALREADY KNOW HOW TO PLAY BASEBALL. WE JUST NEED A TOKEN ADULT AND BETTER EQUIPMENT.
I KNOW! WHY DON'T WE CORK THE BATS?
RIDICULOUS! I COULD REBUILD ALL YOUR EQUIPMENT IN MY LAB FOR PENNIES. ⁝GA-HOY⁝ BUT AS ALBERT EINSTEIN ONCE SAID, "YOU WILL LEARN ABOUT RELATIVITY FASTER THAN I LEARN ABOUT BASEBALL."
WELL, I SUPPOSE YOU'RE RIGHT. I JUST THOUGHT A BRILLIANT MIND LIKE YOURS COULD IMPROVE ON AMERICA'S FAVORITE PASTIME, BUT I GUESS YOU'RE NOT UP TO THE TASK.
NOW SEE HERE, YOUNG BART, IF I CAN OPERATE A SUPER COLLIDER WHILE COMPUTING QUANTUM MECHANICS, I CAN CERTAINLY COACH A BASEBALL TEAM!
NOW SHOW ME YOUR TEAM'S ICE RINK!
YAAAAAY!
YAAAY!

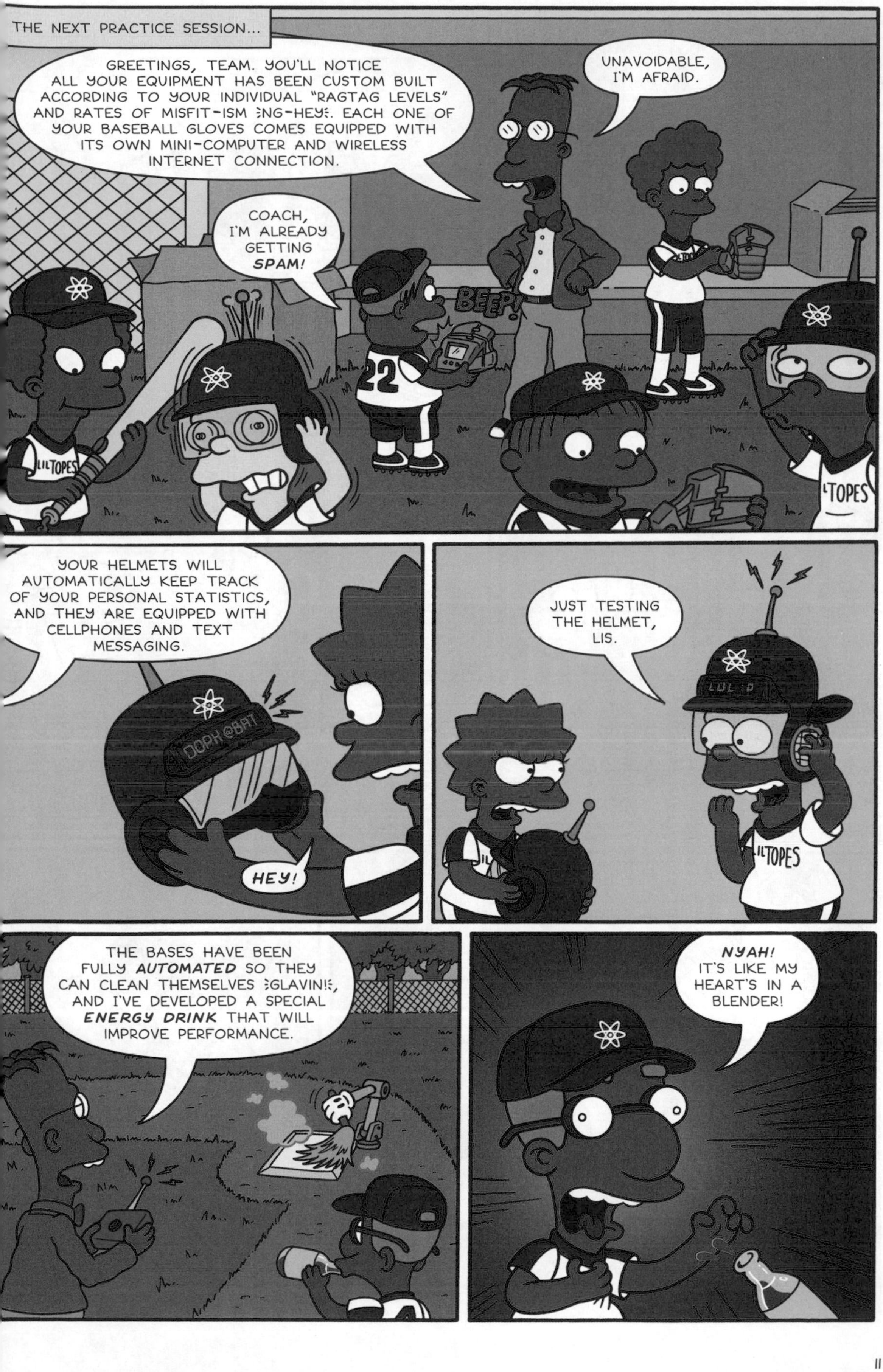

THE NEXT PRACTICE SESSION...
GREETINGS, TEAM. YOU'LL NOTICE ALL YOUR EQUIPMENT HAS BEEN CUSTOM BUILT ACCORDING TO YOUR INDIVIDUAL "RAGTAG LEVELS" AND RATES OF MISFIT-ISM ⋮NG-HEY⋮. EACH ONE OF YOUR BASEBALL GLOVES COMES EQUIPPED WITH ITS OWN MINI-COMPUTER AND WIRELESS INTERNET CONNECTION.
COACH, I'M ALREADY GETTING ***SPAM!***
BEEP!
UNAVOIDABLE, I'M AFRAID.
LIL TOPES
YOUR HELMETS WILL AUTOMATICALLY KEEP TRACK OF YOUR PERSONAL STATISTICS, AND THEY ARE EQUIPPED WITH CELLPHONES AND TEXT MESSAGING.
DOPH @BRT
HEY!
JUST TESTING THE HELMET, LIS.
LIL TOPES
THE BASES HAVE BEEN FULLY ***AUTOMATED*** SO THEY CAN CLEAN THEMSELVES ⋮GLAVIN!⋮, AND I'VE DEVELOPED A SPECIAL ***ENERGY DRINK*** THAT WILL IMPROVE PERFORMANCE.
NYAH! IT'S LIKE MY HEART'S IN A BLENDER!

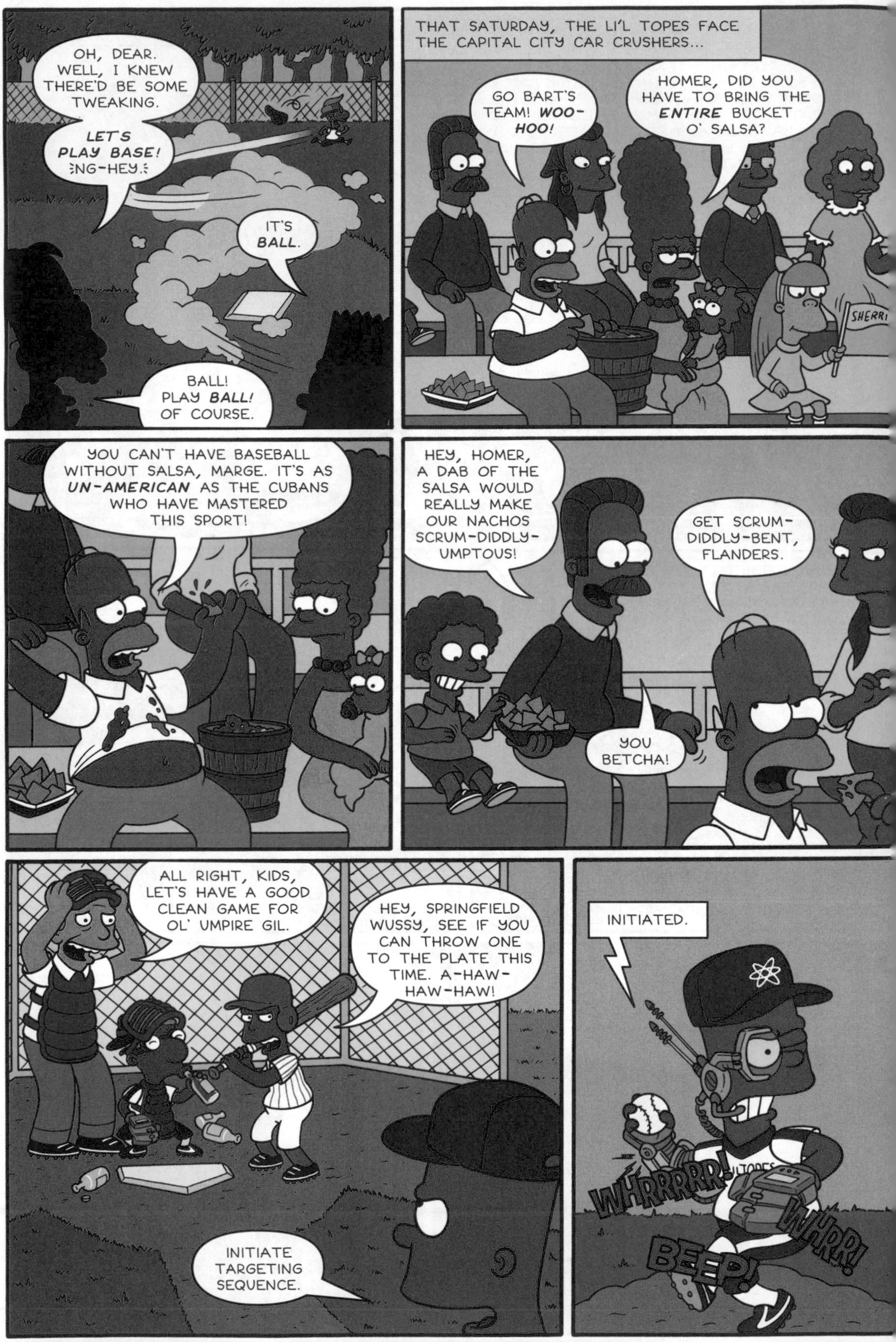
OH, DEAR. WELL, I KNEW THERE'D BE SOME TWEAKING.
LET'S PLAY BASE! ŊNG-HEY.
IT'S BALL.
BALL! PLAY BALL! OF COURSE.
THAT SATURDAY, THE LI'L TOPES FACE THE CAPITAL CITY CAR CRUSHERS...
GO BART'S TEAM! WOO-HOO!
HOMER, DID YOU HAVE TO BRING THE ENTIRE BUCKET O' SALSA?
SHERRI
YOU CAN'T HAVE BASEBALL WITHOUT SALSA, MARGE. IT'S AS UN-AMERICAN AS THE CUBANS WHO HAVE MASTERED THIS SPORT!
HEY, HOMER, A DAB OF THE SALSA WOULD REALLY MAKE OUR NACHOS SCRUM-DIDDLY-UMPTOUS!
GET SCRUM-DIDDLY-BENT, FLANDERS.
YOU BETCHA!
ALL RIGHT, KIDS, LET'S HAVE A GOOD CLEAN GAME FOR OL' UMPIRE GIL.
HEY, SPRINGFIELD WUSSY, SEE IF YOU CAN THROW ONE TO THE PLATE THIS TIME. A-HAW-HAW-HAW!
INITIATE TARGETING SEQUENCE.
INITIATED.
WHRRRRR!
WHRR!
BEEP!

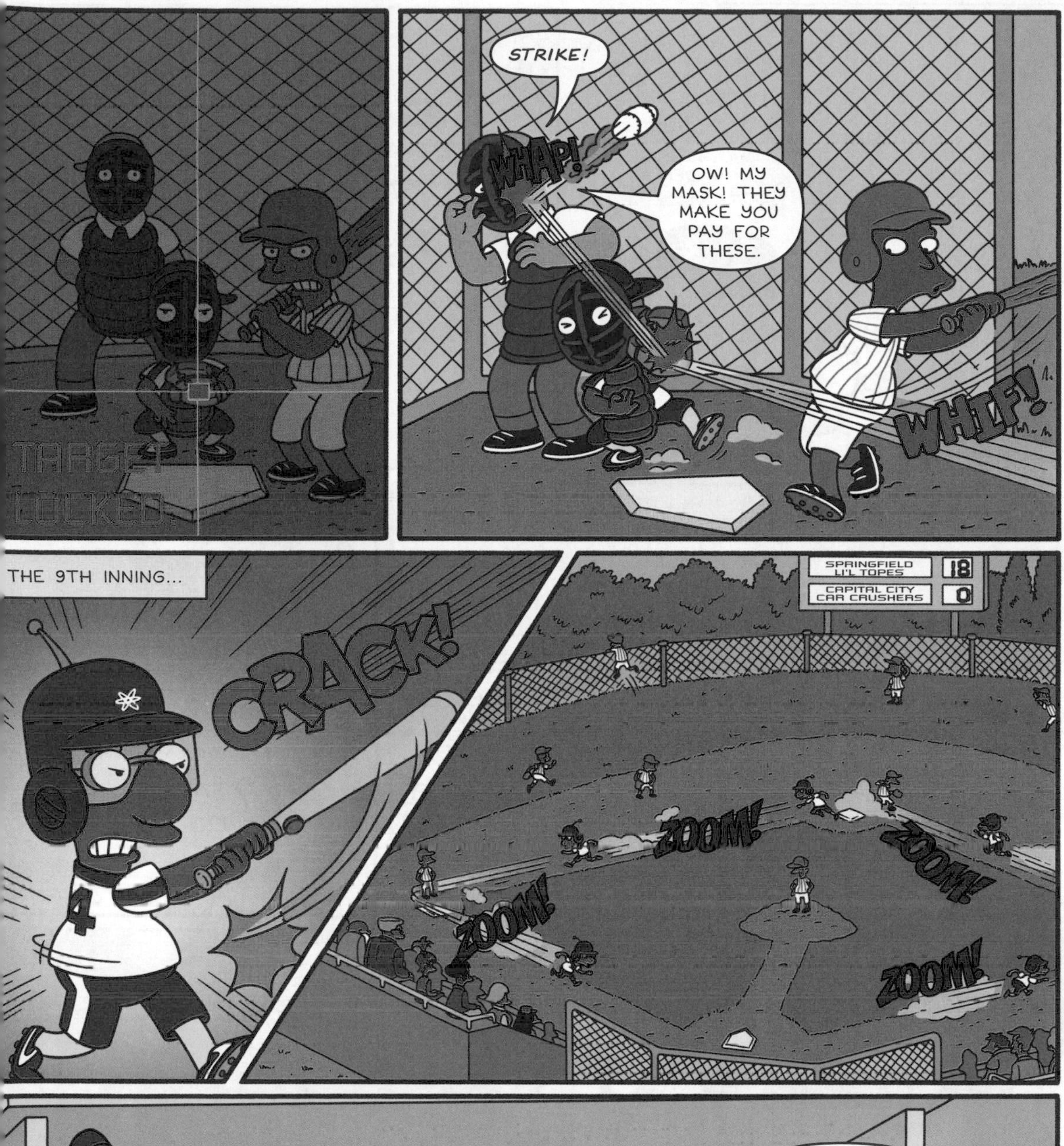
TARGET LOCKED.
STRIKE!
WHAP!
OW! MY MASK! THEY MAKE YOU PAY FOR THESE.
WHIF!
THE 9TH INNING...
CRACK!
SPRINGFIELD LI'L TOPES 18
CAPITAL CITY CAR CRUSHERS 0
ZOOM!
ZOOM!
ZOOM!
ZOOM!
NICE HIT, MILHOUSE! WE WON!
YEAH-YEAH-YEAH! W-WHERE'S MY ENERGY DRINK?

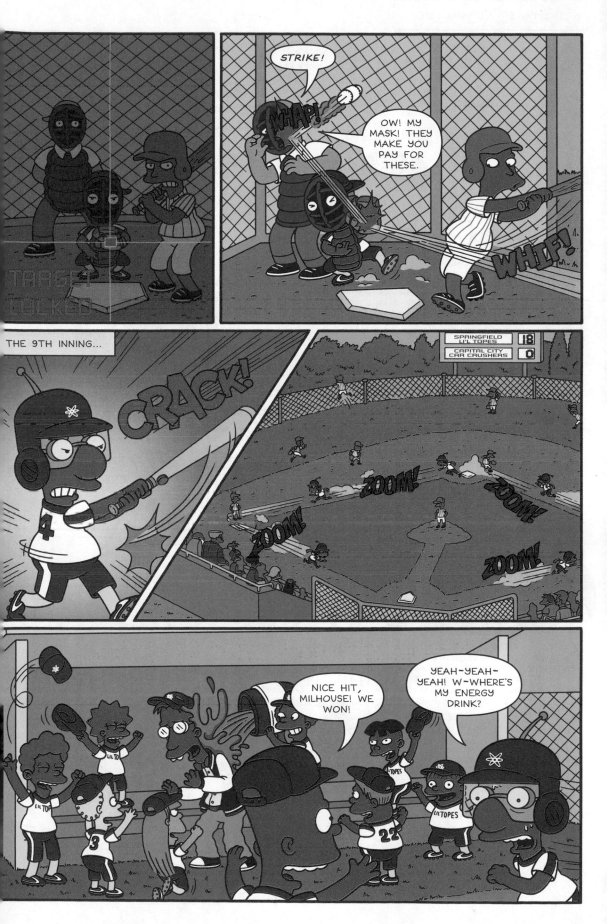

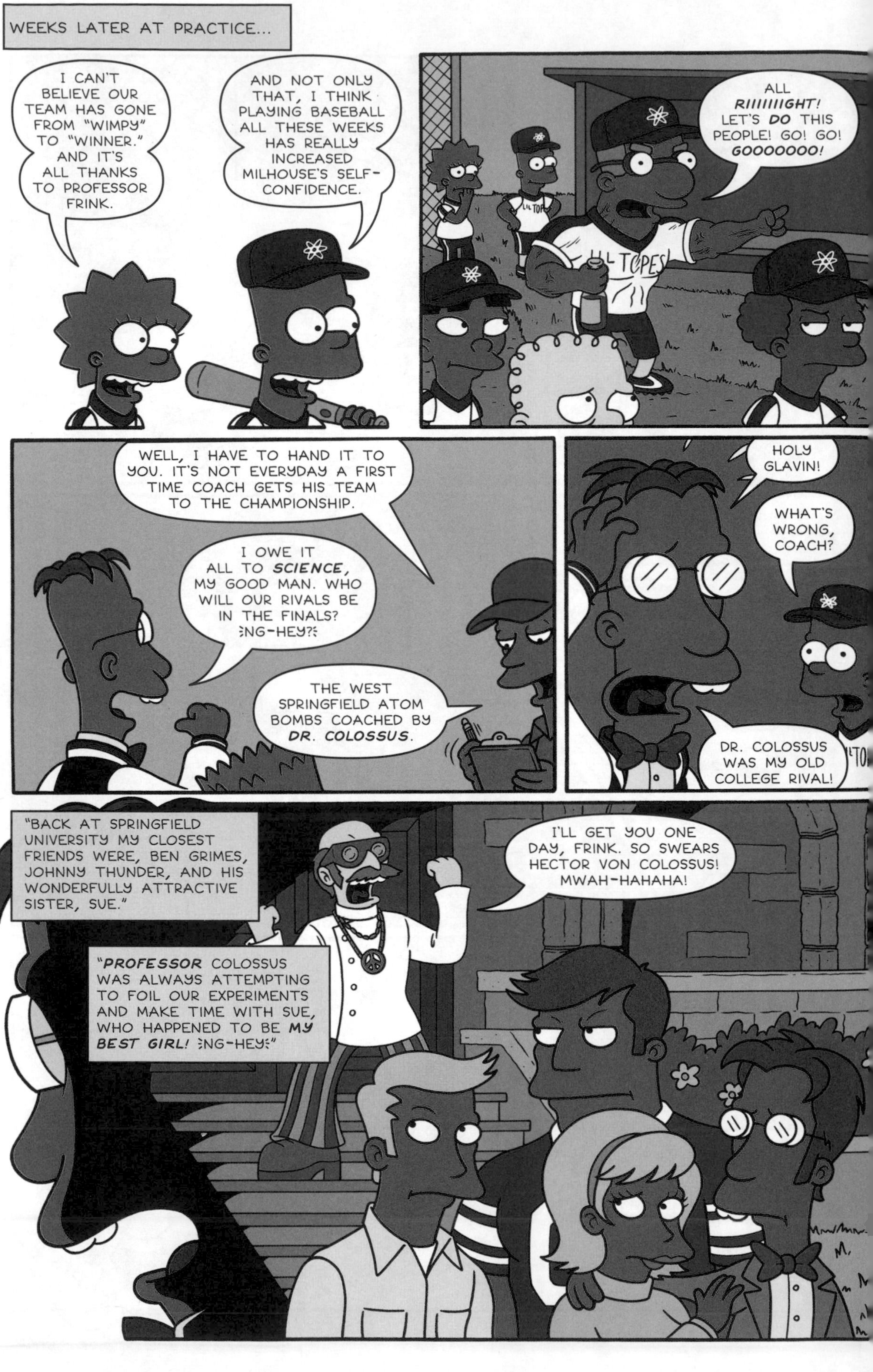
WEEKS LATER AT PRACTICE...
I CAN'T BELIEVE OUR TEAM HAS GONE FROM "WIMPY" TO "WINNER." AND IT'S ALL THANKS TO PROFESSOR FRINK.
AND NOT ONLY THAT, I THINK PLAYING BASEBALL ALL THESE WEEKS HAS REALLY INCREASED MILHOUSE'S SELF-CONFIDENCE.
ALL RIIIIIIIGHT! LET'S DO THIS PEOPLE! GO! GO! GOOOOOOO!
WELL, I HAVE TO HAND IT TO YOU. IT'S NOT EVERYDAY A FIRST TIME COACH GETS HIS TEAM TO THE CHAMPIONSHIP.
I OWE IT ALL TO SCIENCE, MY GOOD MAN. WHO WILL OUR RIVALS BE IN THE FINALS? NG-HEY?
THE WEST SPRINGFIELD ATOM BOMBS COACHED BY DR. COLOSSUS.
HOLY GLAVIN!
WHAT'S WRONG, COACH?
DR. COLOSSUS WAS MY OLD COLLEGE RIVAL!
"BACK AT SPRINGFIELD UNIVERSITY MY CLOSEST FRIENDS WERE, BEN GRIMES, JOHNNY THUNDER, AND HIS WONDERFULLY ATTRACTIVE SISTER, SUE."
I'LL GET YOU ONE DAY, FRINK. SO SWEARS HECTOR VON COLOSSUS! MWAH-HAHAHA!
"PROFESSOR COLOSSUS WAS ALWAYS ATTEMPTING TO FOIL OUR EXPERIMENTS AND MAKE TIME WITH SUE, WHO HAPPENED TO BE MY BEST GIRL! NG-HEY"

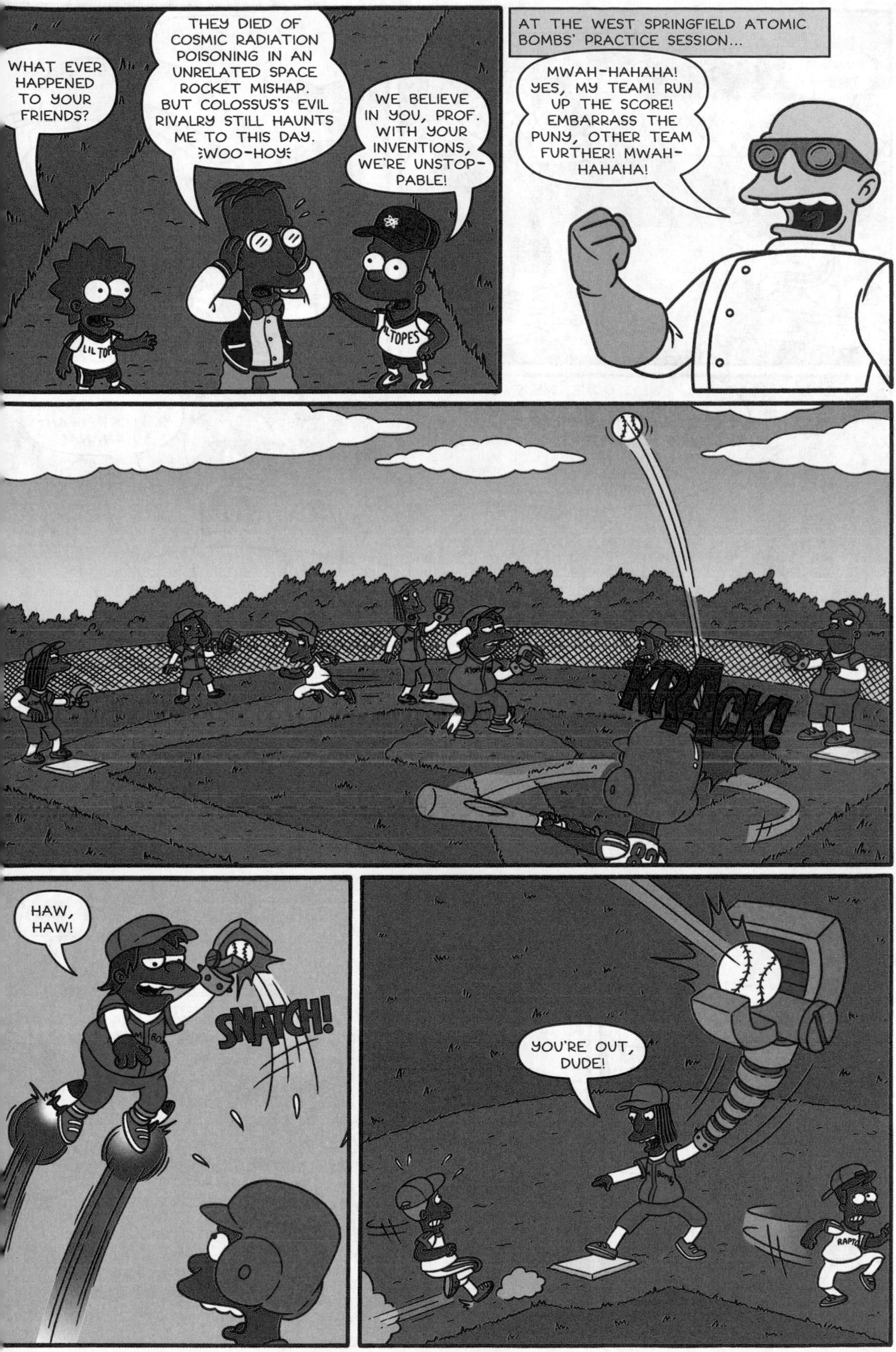

WHAT EVER HAPPENED TO YOUR FRIENDS?
THEY DIED OF COSMIC RADIATION POISONING IN AN UNRELATED SPACE ROCKET MISHAP. BUT COLOSSUS'S EVIL RIVALRY STILL HAUNTS ME TO THIS DAY. WOO-HOY
WE BELIEVE IN YOU, PROF. WITH YOUR INVENTIONS, WE'RE UNSTOP-PABLE!
LIL TOPES
LIL TOPES
AT THE WEST SPRINGFIELD ATOMIC BOMBS' PRACTICE SESSION...
MWAH-HAHAHA! YES, MY TEAM! RUN UP THE SCORE! EMBARRASS THE PUNY, OTHER TEAM FURTHER! MWAH-HAHAHA!
KRACK!
HAW, HAW!
SNATCH!
YOU'RE OUT, DUDE!

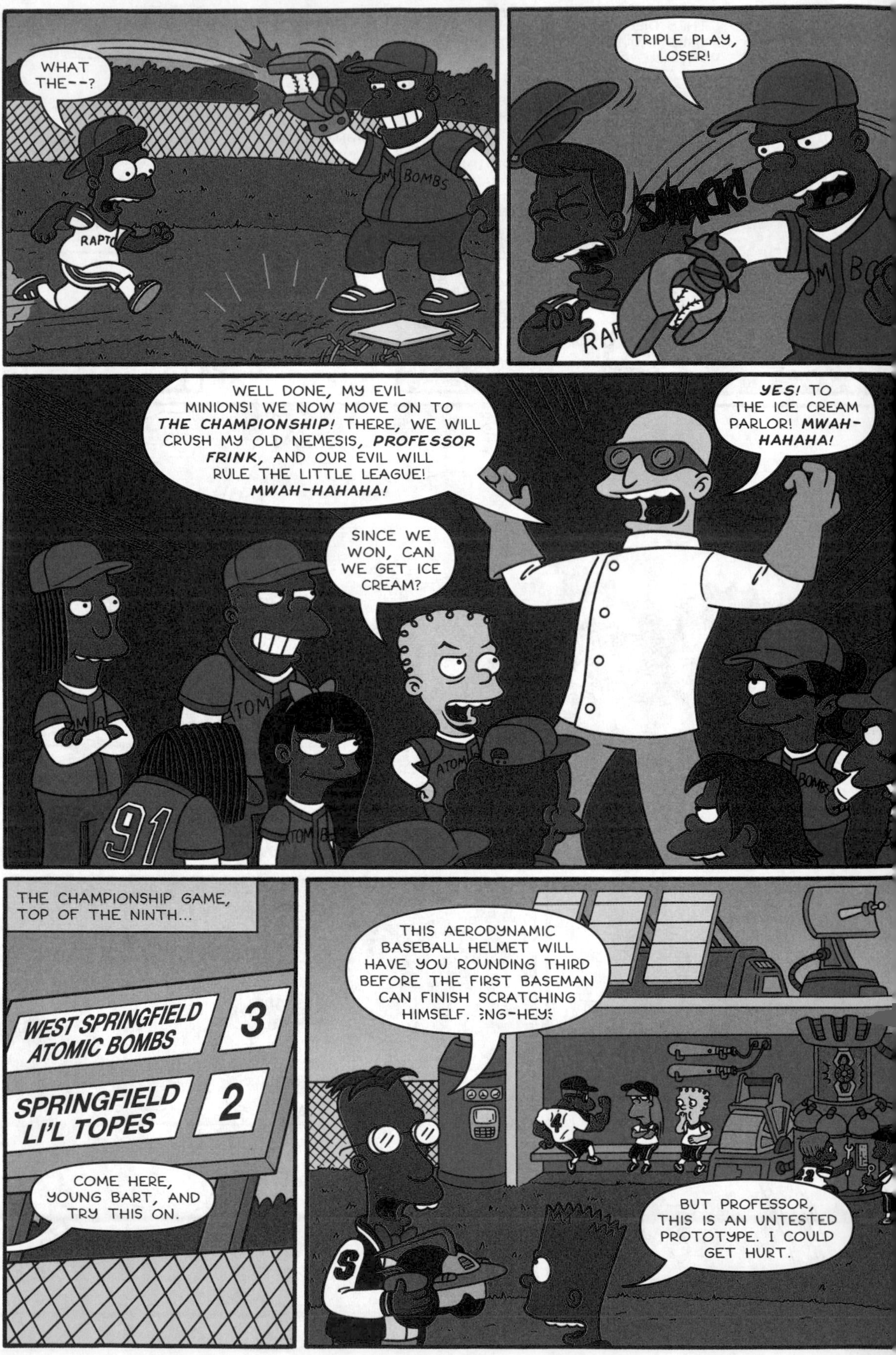
WHAT THE--?
TRIPLE PLAY, LOSER!
SMACK!
WELL DONE, MY EVIL MINIONS! WE NOW MOVE ON TO THE CHAMPIONSHIP! THERE, WE WILL CRUSH MY OLD NEMESIS, PROFESSOR FRINK, AND OUR EVIL WILL RULE THE LITTLE LEAGUE! MWAH-HAHAHA!
YES! TO THE ICE CREAM PARLOR! MWAH-HAHAHA!
SINCE WE WON, CAN WE GET ICE CREAM?
THE CHAMPIONSHIP GAME, TOP OF THE NINTH...
WEST SPRINGFIELD ATOMIC BOMBS 3
SPRINGFIELD LI'L TOPES 2
COME HERE, YOUNG BART, AND TRY THIS ON.
THIS AERODYNAMIC BASEBALL HELMET WILL HAVE YOU ROUNDING THIRD BEFORE THE FIRST BASEMAN CAN FINISH SCRATCHING HIMSELF. NG-HEY
BUT PROFESSOR, THIS IS AN UNTESTED PROTOTYPE. I COULD GET HURT.

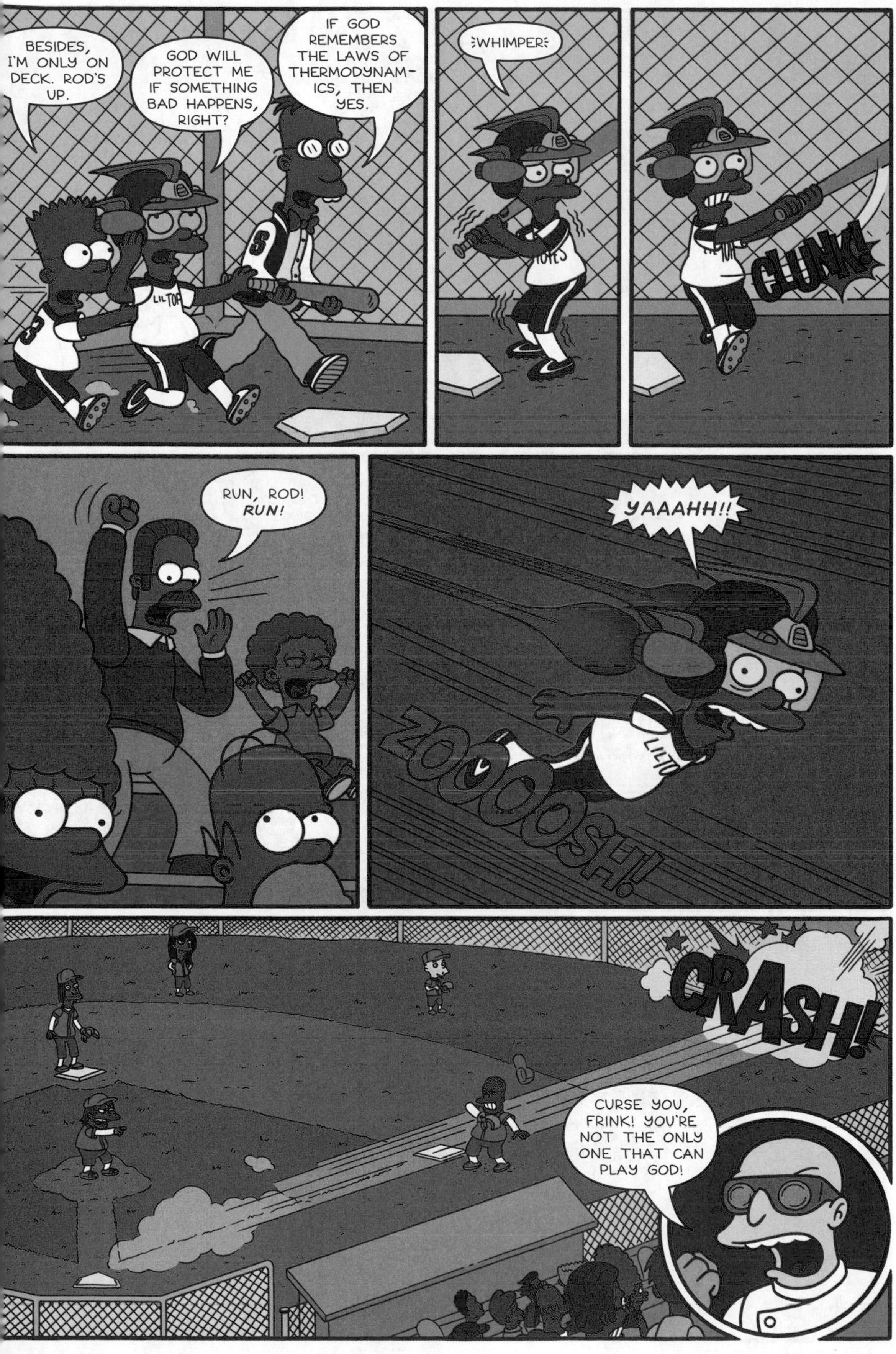
BESIDES, I'M ONLY ON DECK. ROD'S UP.
GOD WILL PROTECT ME IF SOMETHING BAD HAPPENS, RIGHT?
IF GOD REMEMBERS THE LAWS OF THERMODYNAMICS, THEN YES.
WHIMPER
CLUNK!
RUN, ROD! *RUN!*
YAAAHH!!
ZOOOOSH!!
CRASH!
CURSE YOU, FRINK! YOU'RE NOT THE ONLY ONE THAT CAN PLAY GOD!

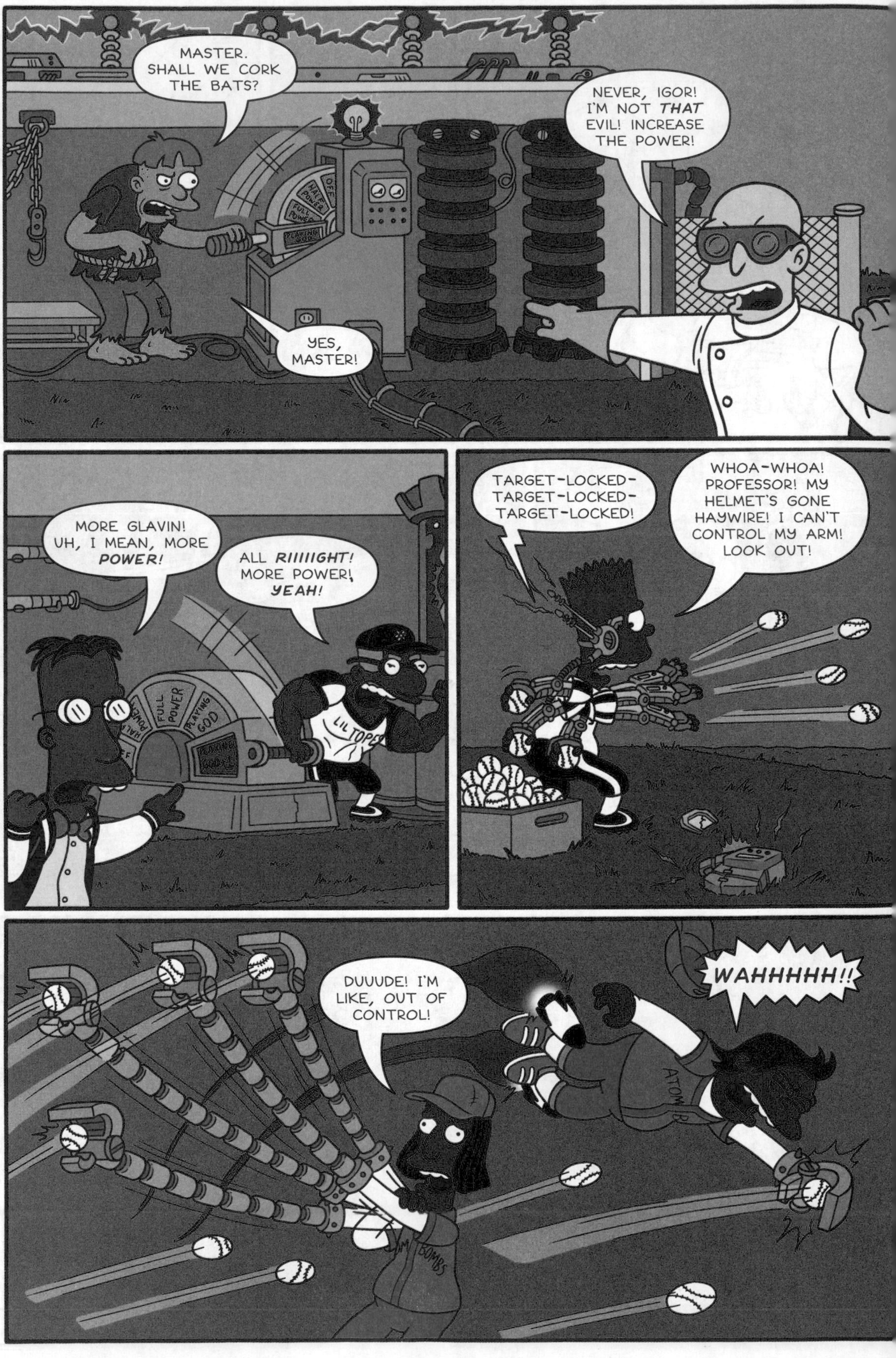
MASTER. SHALL WE CORK THE BATS?
NEVER, IGOR! I'M NOT *THAT* EVIL! INCREASE THE POWER!
YES, MASTER!
MORE GLAVIN! UH, I MEAN, MORE *POWER!*
ALL *RIIIIIGHT!* MORE POWER! *YEAH!*
TARGET-LOCKED- TARGET-LOCKED- TARGET-LOCKED!
WHOA-WHOA! PROFESSOR! MY HELMET'S GONE HAYWIRE! I CAN'T CONTROL MY ARM! LOOK OUT!
DUUUDE! I'M LIKE, OUT OF CONTROL!
WAHHHHH!!

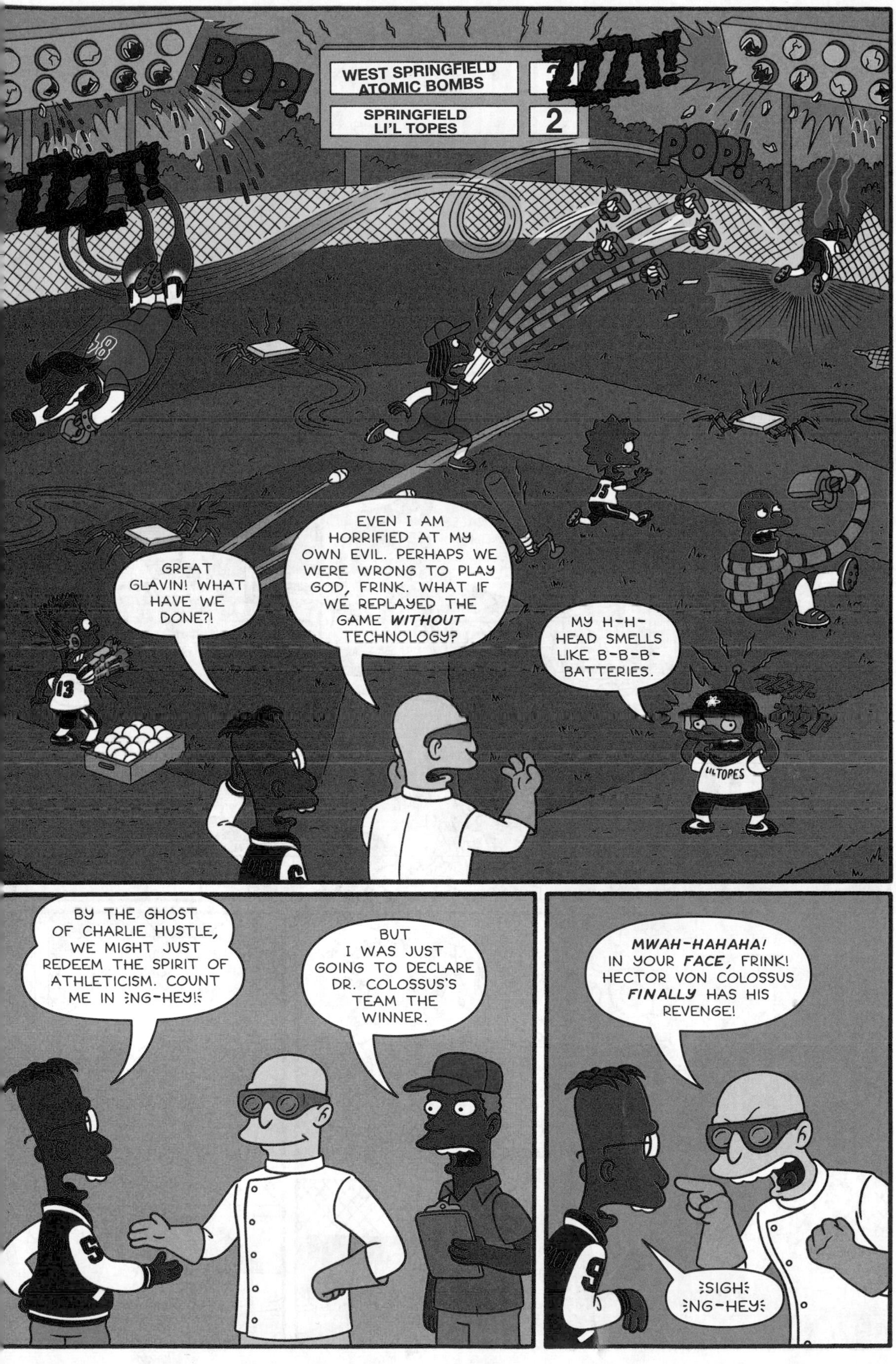
WEST SPRINGFIELD ATOMIC BOMBS
SPRINGFIELD LI'L TOPES 2
POP!
ZZZT!
ZZZT!
POP!
GREAT GLAVIN! WHAT HAVE WE DONE?!
EVEN I AM HORRIFIED AT MY OWN EVIL. PERHAPS WE WERE WRONG TO PLAY GOD, FRINK. WHAT IF WE REPLAYED THE GAME ***WITHOUT*** TECHNOLOGY?
MY H-H-HEAD SMELLS LIKE B-B-B-BATTERIES.
LI'L TOPES
BY THE GHOST OF CHARLIE HUSTLE, WE MIGHT JUST REDEEM THE SPIRIT OF ATHLETICISM. COUNT ME IN ⁝NG-HEY!⁝
BUT I WAS JUST GOING TO DECLARE DR. COLOSSUS'S TEAM THE WINNER.
MWAH-HAHAHA! IN YOUR ***FACE,*** FRINK! HECTOR VON COLOSSUS ***FINALLY*** HAS HIS REVENGE!
⁝SIGH⁝ ⁝NG-HEY⁝

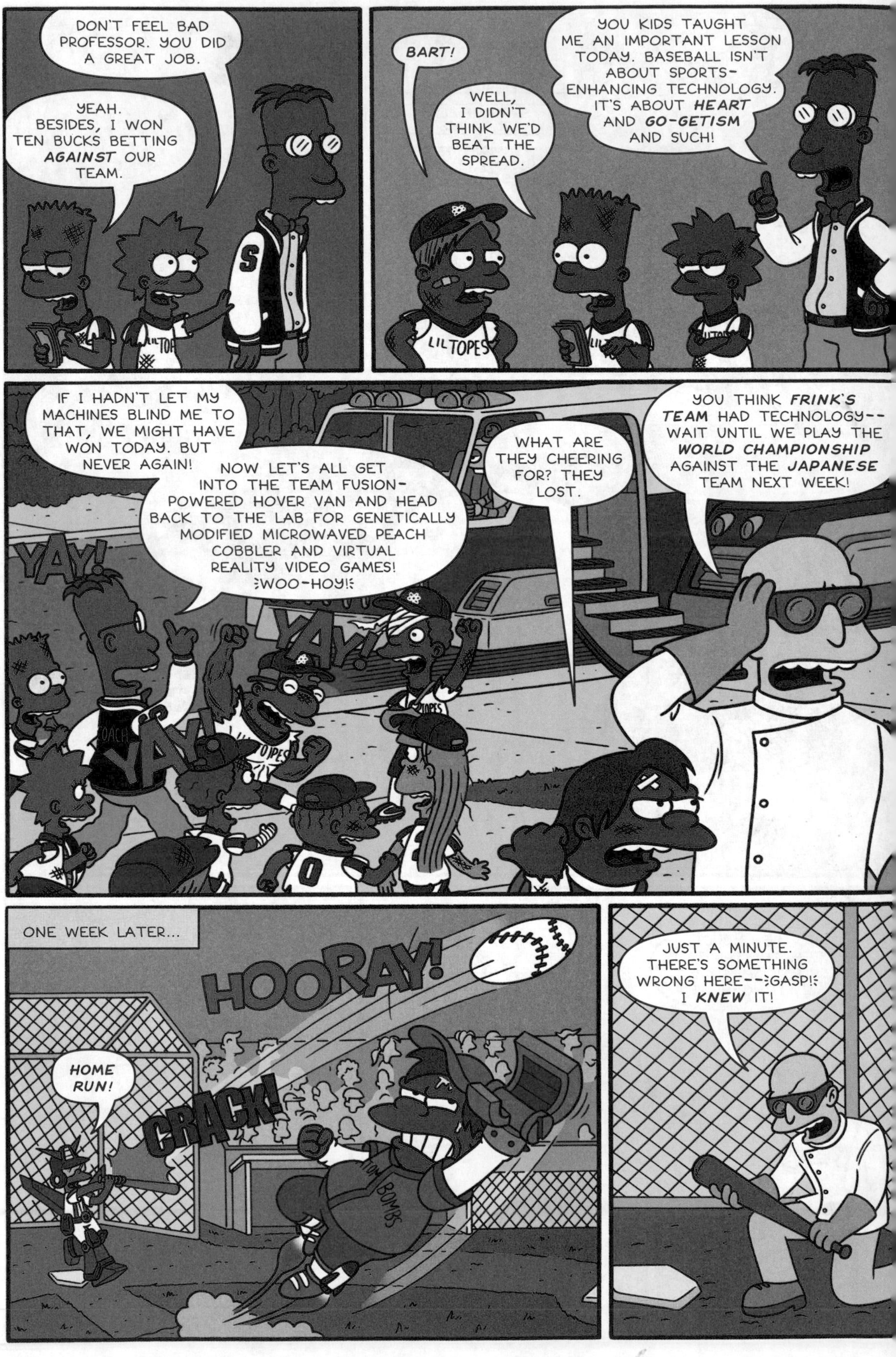
DON'T FEEL BAD PROFESSOR. YOU DID A GREAT JOB.
YEAH. BESIDES, I WON TEN BUCKS BETTING AGAINST OUR TEAM.
BART!
WELL, I DIDN'T THINK WE'D BEAT THE SPREAD.
YOU KIDS TAUGHT ME AN IMPORTANT LESSON TODAY. BASEBALL ISN'T ABOUT SPORTS-ENHANCING TECHNOLOGY. IT'S ABOUT HEART AND GO-GETISM AND SUCH!
IF I HADN'T LET MY MACHINES BLIND ME TO THAT, WE MIGHT HAVE WON TODAY. BUT NEVER AGAIN!
NOW LET'S ALL GET INTO THE TEAM FUSION-POWERED HOVER VAN AND HEAD BACK TO THE LAB FOR GENETICALLY MODIFIED MICROWAVED PEACH COBBLER AND VIRTUAL REALITY VIDEO GAMES! WOO-HOY!
YAY!
YAY!
YAY!
WHAT ARE THEY CHEERING FOR? THEY LOST.
YOU THINK FRINK'S TEAM HAD TECHNOLOGY--WAIT UNTIL WE PLAY THE WORLD CHAMPIONSHIP AGAINST THE JAPANESE TEAM NEXT WEEK!
ONE WEEK LATER...
HOORAY!
HOME RUN!
CRACK!
JUST A MINUTE. THERE'S SOMETHING WRONG HERE--GASP! I KNEW IT!

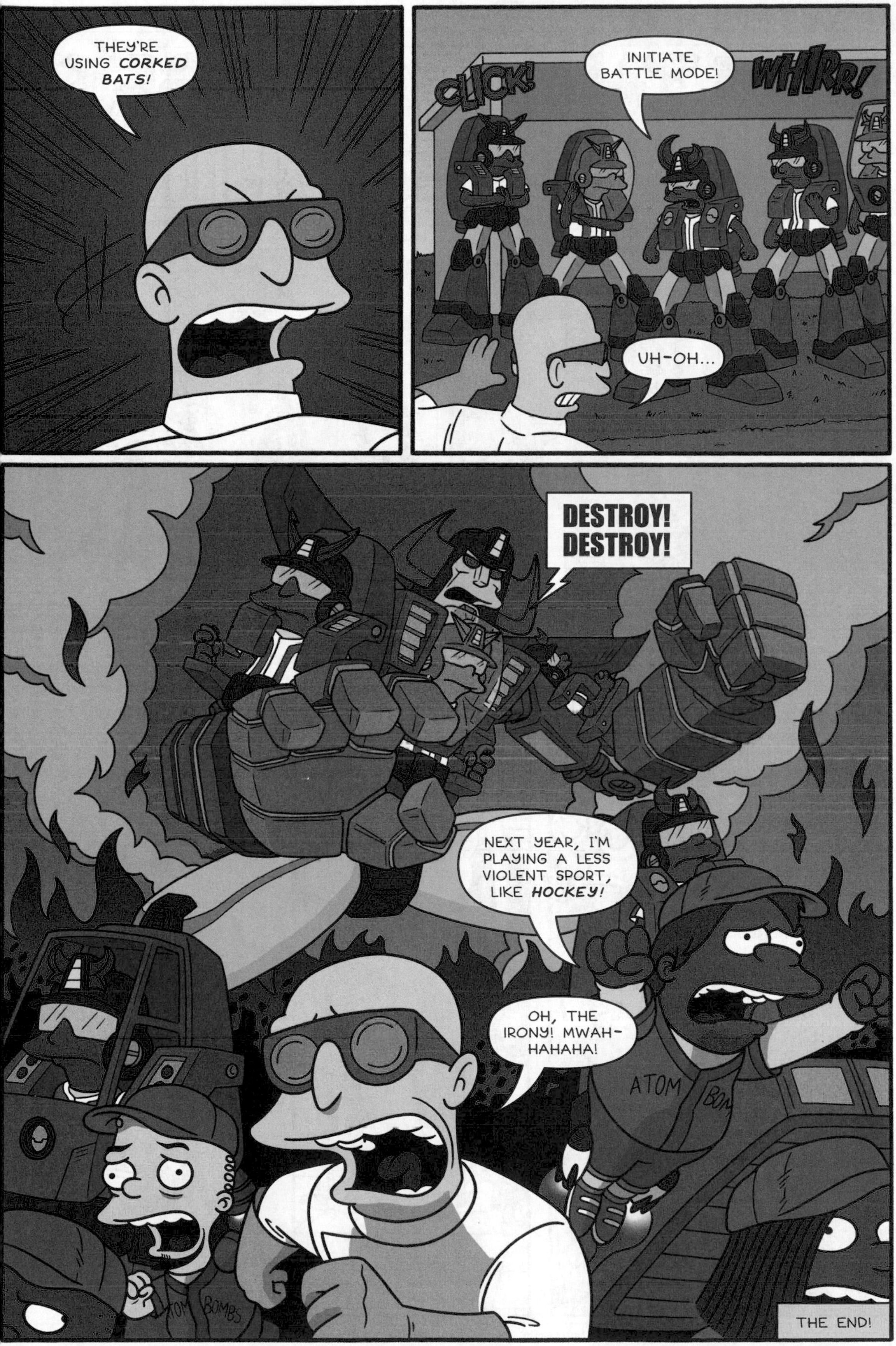
THEY'RE USING *CORKED BATS!*
INITIATE BATTLE MODE!
CLICK!
WHIRR!
UH-OH...
DESTROY! DESTROY!
NEXT YEAR, I'M PLAYING A LESS VIOLENT SPORT, LIKE *HOCKEY!*
OH, THE IRONY! MWAH-HAHAHA!
ATOM BOMBS
THE END!

TONY DIGEROLAMO WRITER | *JASON HO* PENCILS | *MIKE ROTE* INKS | *NATHAN HAMILL* COLORS | *KAREN BATES* LETTERS | *BILL MORRISON* EDITOR

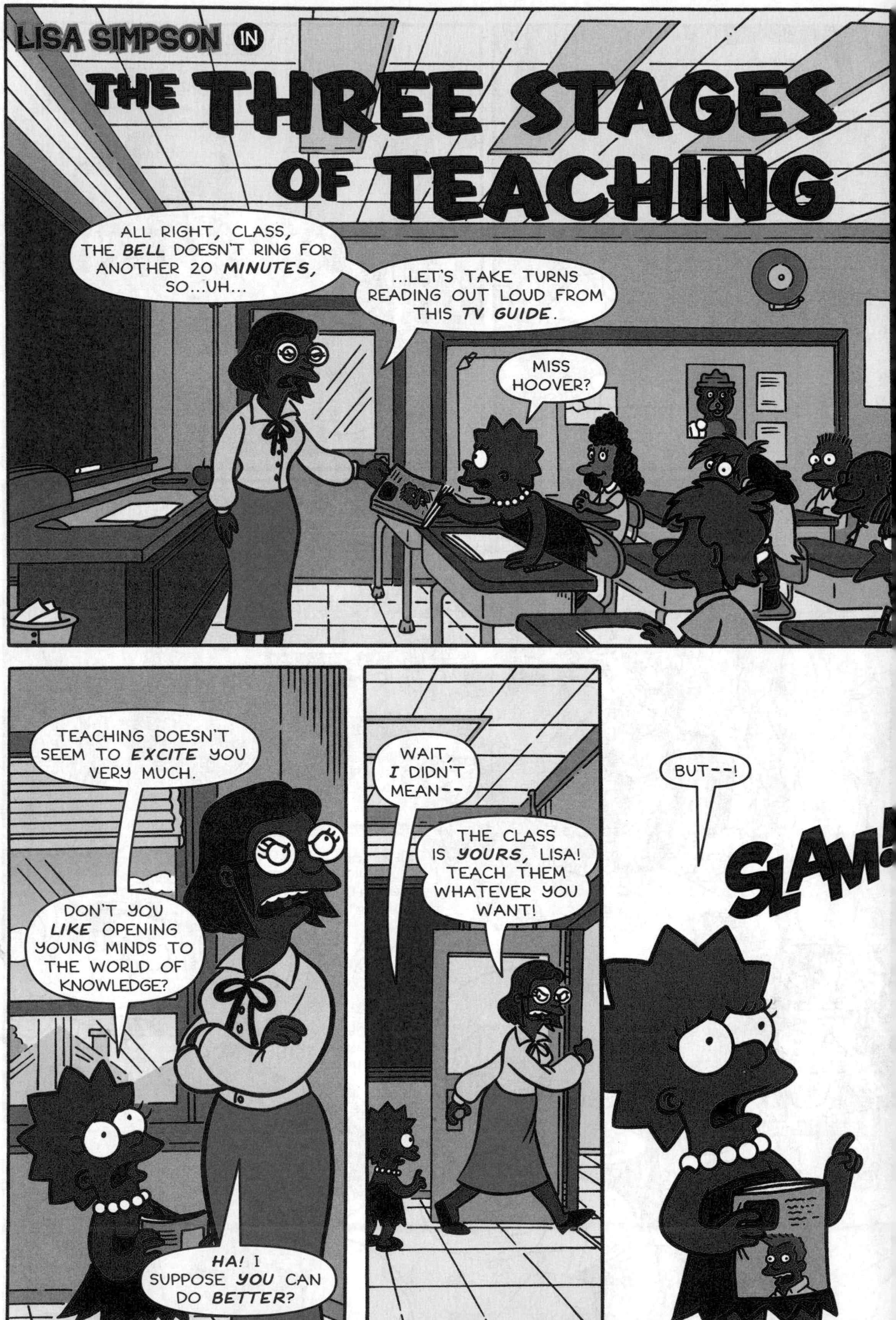
LISA SIMPSON IN
THE THREE STAGES OF TEACHING
ALL RIGHT, CLASS, THE BELL DOESN'T RING FOR ANOTHER 20 MINUTES, SO...UH...
...LET'S TAKE TURNS READING OUT LOUD FROM THIS TV GUIDE.
MISS HOOVER?
TEACHING DOESN'T SEEM TO EXCITE YOU VERY MUCH.
DON'T YOU LIKE OPENING YOUNG MINDS TO THE WORLD OF KNOWLEDGE?
HA! I SUPPOSE YOU CAN DO BETTER?
WAIT, I DIDN'T MEAN--
THE CLASS IS YOURS, LISA! TEACH THEM WHATEVER YOU WANT!
BUT--!
SLAM!

TOM PEYER WRITER | *JOHN DELANEY* PENCILS | *HOWARD SHUM* INKS | *ART VILLANUEVA* COLORS | *CHRIS UNGAR* LETTERS | *BILL MORRISON* EDITOR

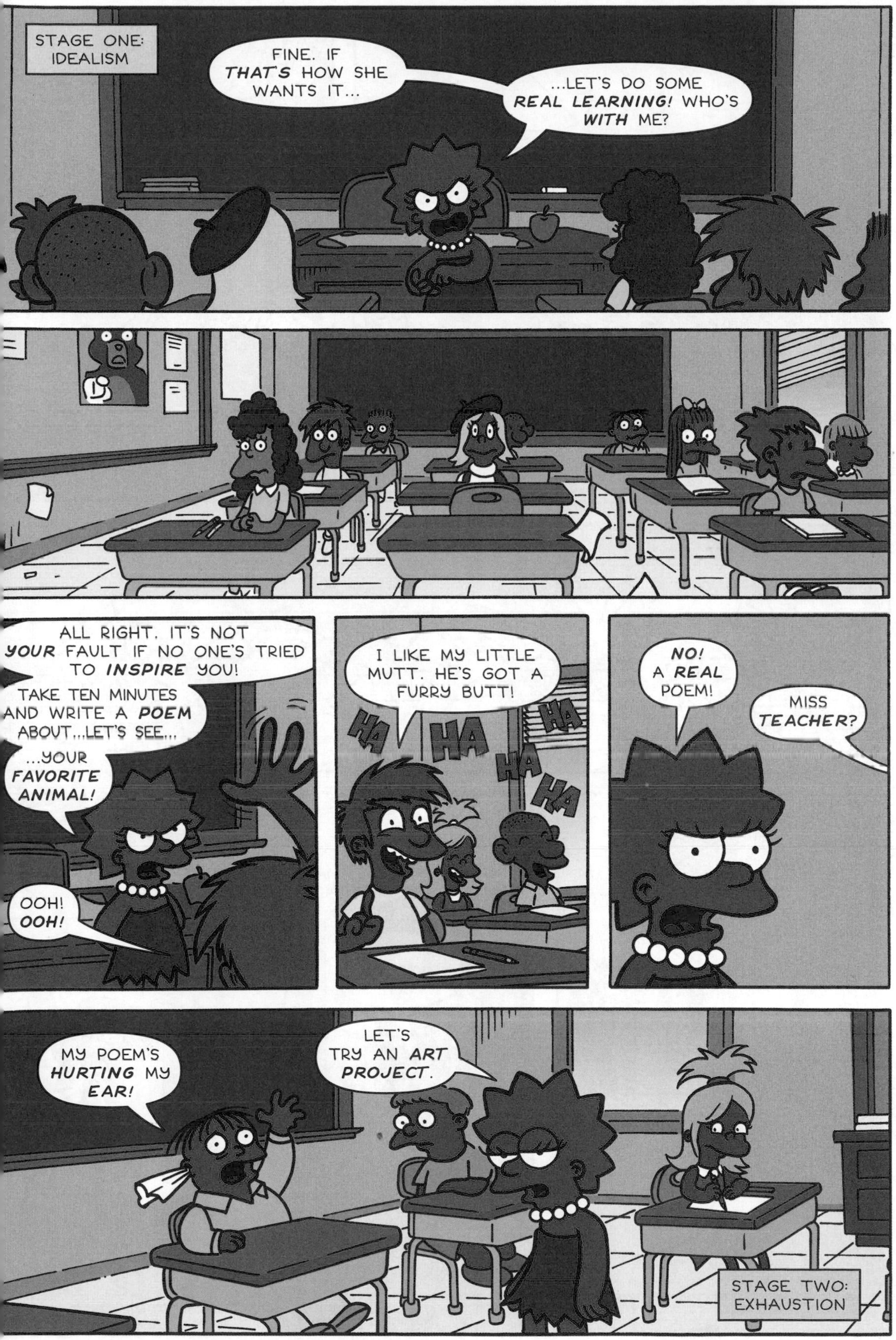
STAGE ONE: IDEALISM
FINE. IF THAT'S HOW SHE WANTS IT...
...LET'S DO SOME REAL LEARNING! WHO'S WITH ME?
ALL RIGHT. IT'S NOT YOUR FAULT IF NO ONE'S TRIED TO INSPIRE YOU!
TAKE TEN MINUTES AND WRITE A POEM ABOUT...LET'S SEE...
...YOUR FAVORITE ANIMAL!
OOH! OOH!
I LIKE MY LITTLE MUTT. HE'S GOT A FURRY BUTT!
HA HA HA HA HA
NO! A REAL POEM!
MISS TEACHER?
MY POEM'S HURTING MY EAR!
LET'S TRY AN ART PROJECT.
STAGE TWO: EXHAUSTION

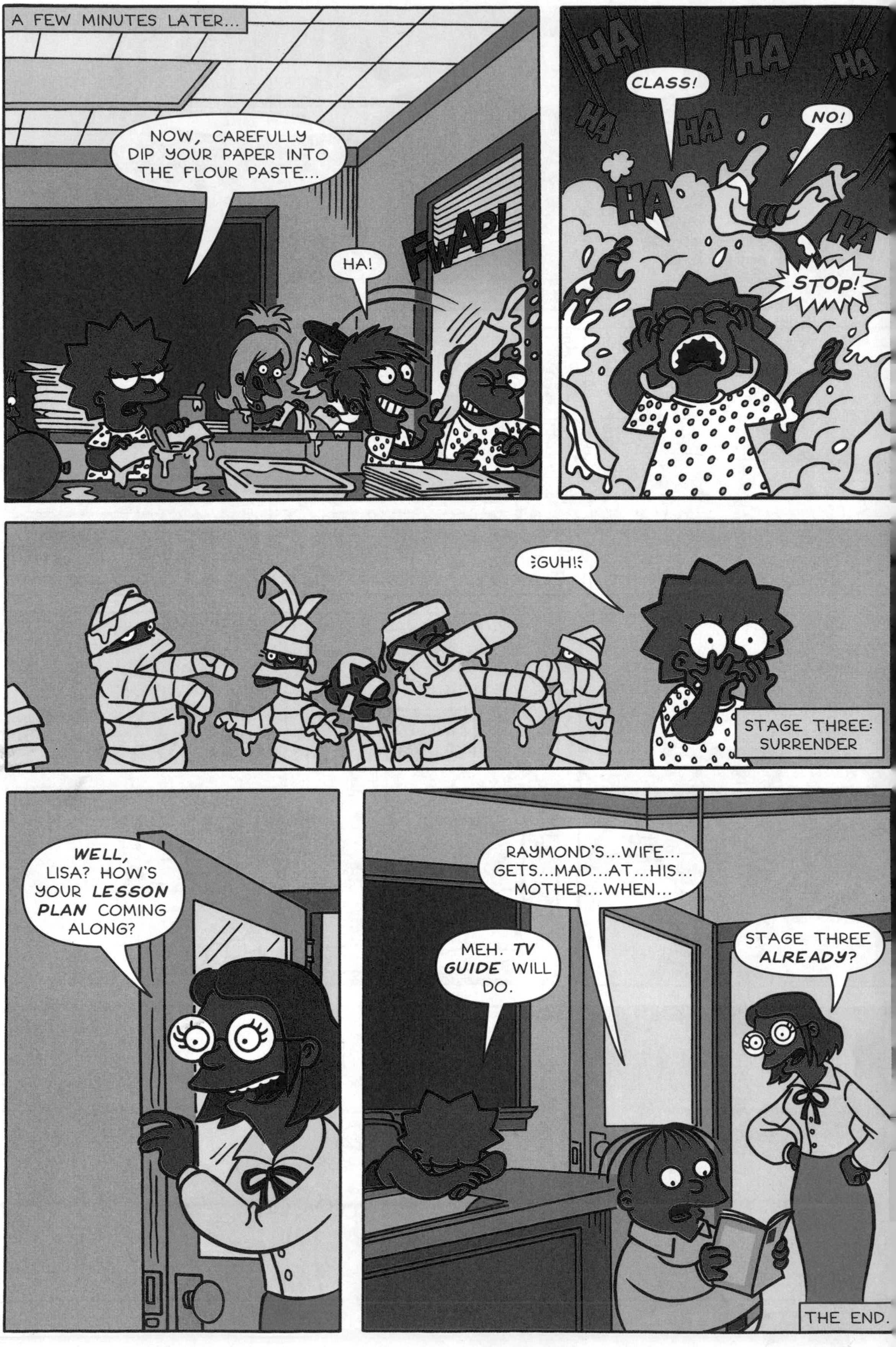
A FEW MINUTES LATER...
NOW, CAREFULLY DIP YOUR PAPER INTO THE FLOUR PASTE...
HA!
FWAP!
HA HA HA HA HA HA HA
CLASS!
NO!
STOP!
GUH!
STAGE THREE: SURRENDER
WELL, LISA? HOW'S YOUR LESSON PLAN COMING ALONG?
RAYMOND'S...WIFE... GETS...MAD...AT...HIS... MOTHER...WHEN...
MEH. TV GUIDE WILL DO.
STAGE THREE ALREADY?
THE END.

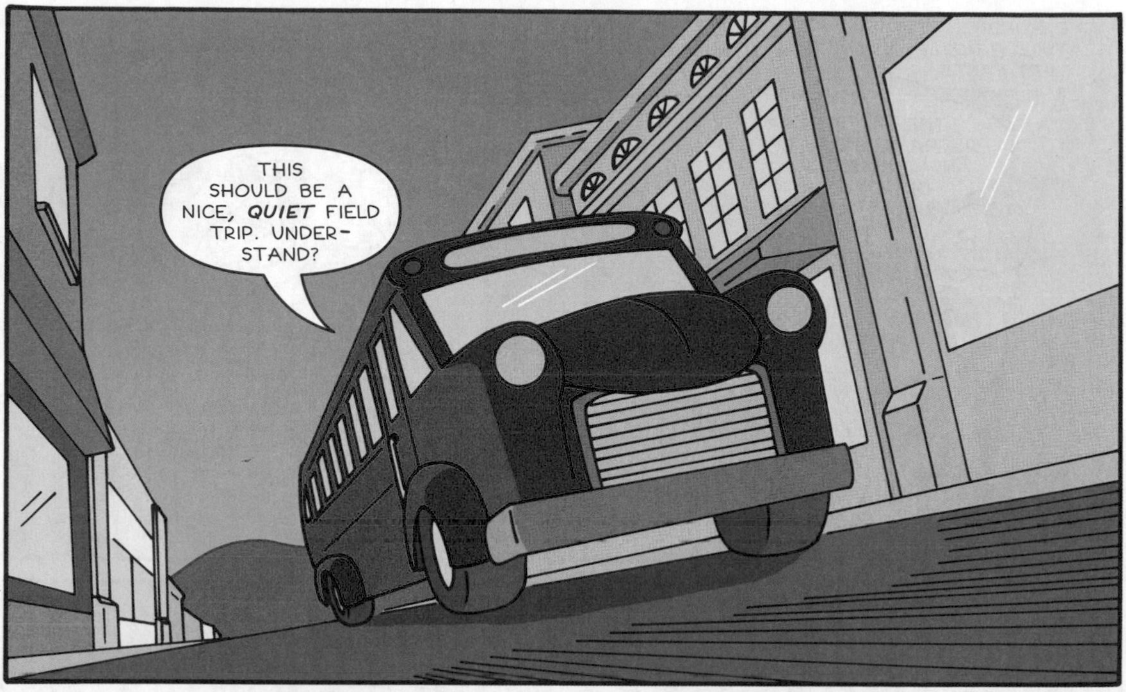
THIS SHOULD BE A NICE, ***QUIET*** FIELD TRIP. UNDER-STAND?

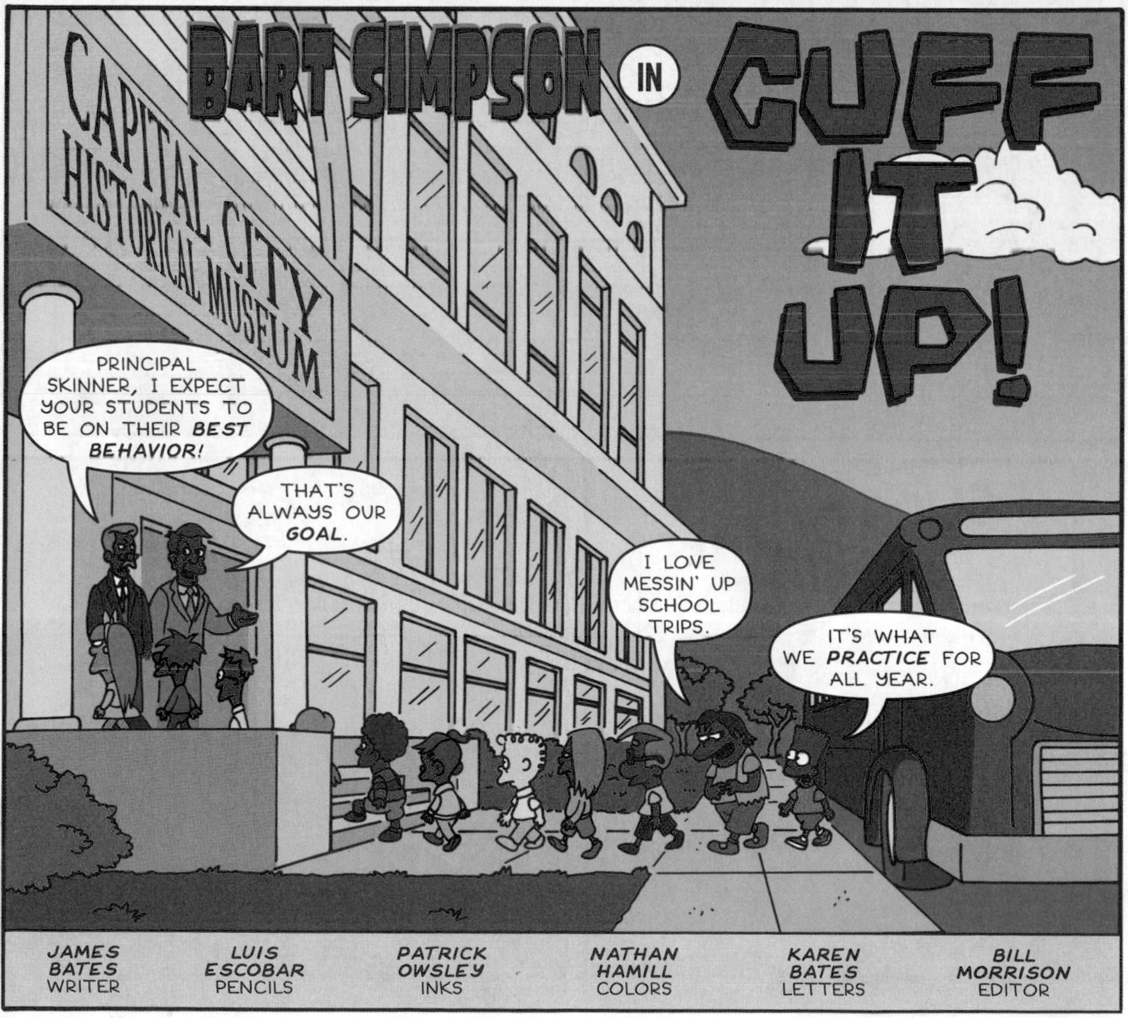
BART SIMPSON IN
CUFF IT UP!
CAPITAL CITY HISTORICAL MUSEUM
PRINCIPAL SKINNER, I EXPECT YOUR STUDENTS TO BE ON THEIR ***BEST BEHAVIOR!***
THAT'S ALWAYS OUR ***GOAL***.
I LOVE MESSIN' UP SCHOOL TRIPS.
IT'S WHAT WE ***PRACTICE*** FOR ALL YEAR.

JAMES BATES WRITER

LUIS ESCOBAR PENCILS

PATRICK OWSLEY INKS

NATHAN HAMILL COLORS

KAREN BATES LETTERS

BILL MORRISON EDITOR

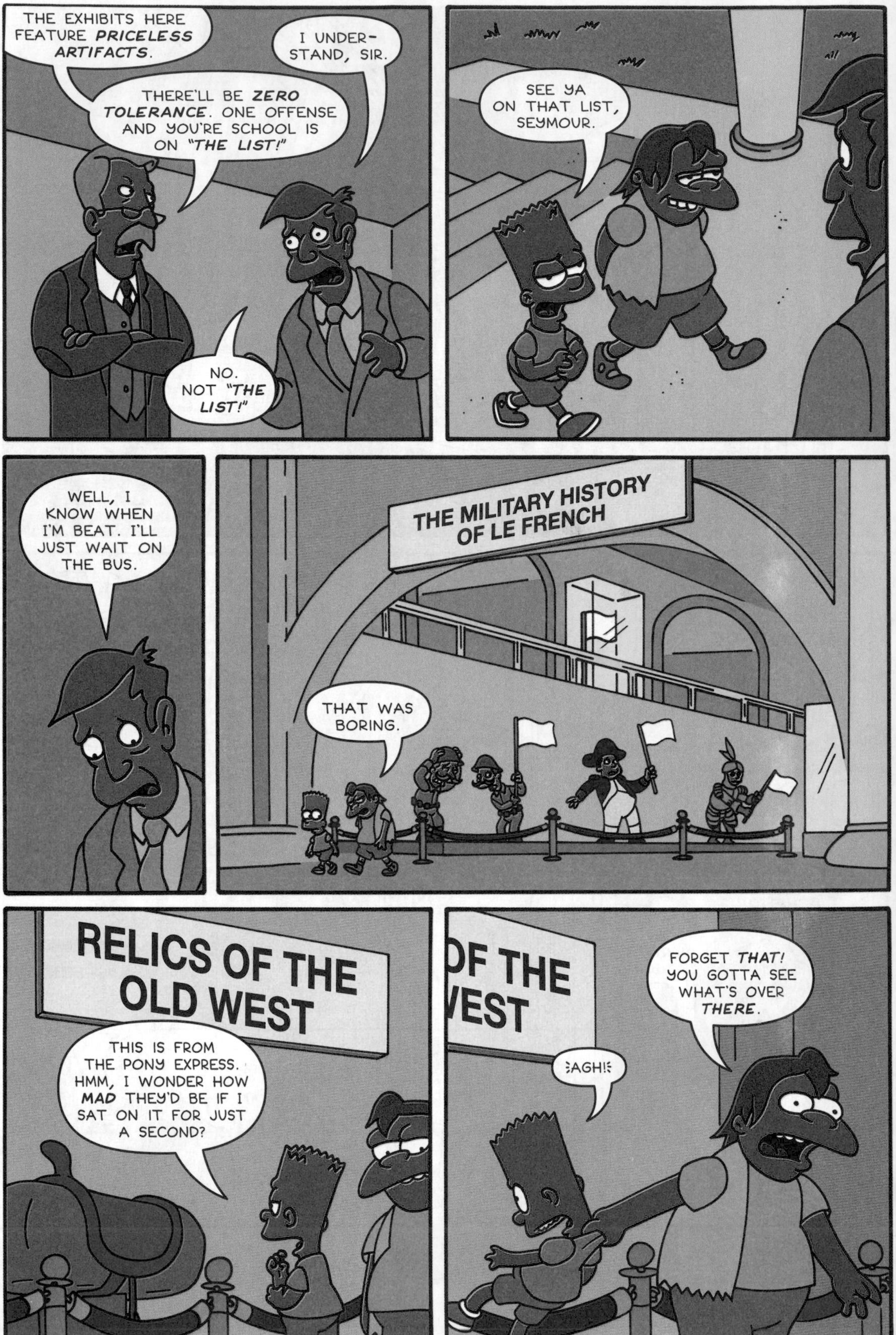
THE EXHIBITS HERE FEATURE PRICELESS ARTIFACTS.
THERE'LL BE ZERO TOLERANCE. ONE OFFENSE AND YOU'RE SCHOOL IS ON "THE LIST!"
I UNDER-STAND, SIR.
NO. NOT "THE LIST!"
SEE YA ON THAT LIST, SEYMOUR.
WELL, I KNOW WHEN I'M BEAT. I'LL JUST WAIT ON THE BUS.
THE MILITARY HISTORY OF LE FRENCH
THAT WAS BORING.
RELICS OF THE OLD WEST
THIS IS FROM THE PONY EXPRESS. HMM, I WONDER HOW MAD THEY'D BE IF I SAT ON IT FOR JUST A SECOND?
OF THE WEST
FORGET THAT! YOU GOTTA SEE WHAT'S OVER THERE.
AGH!

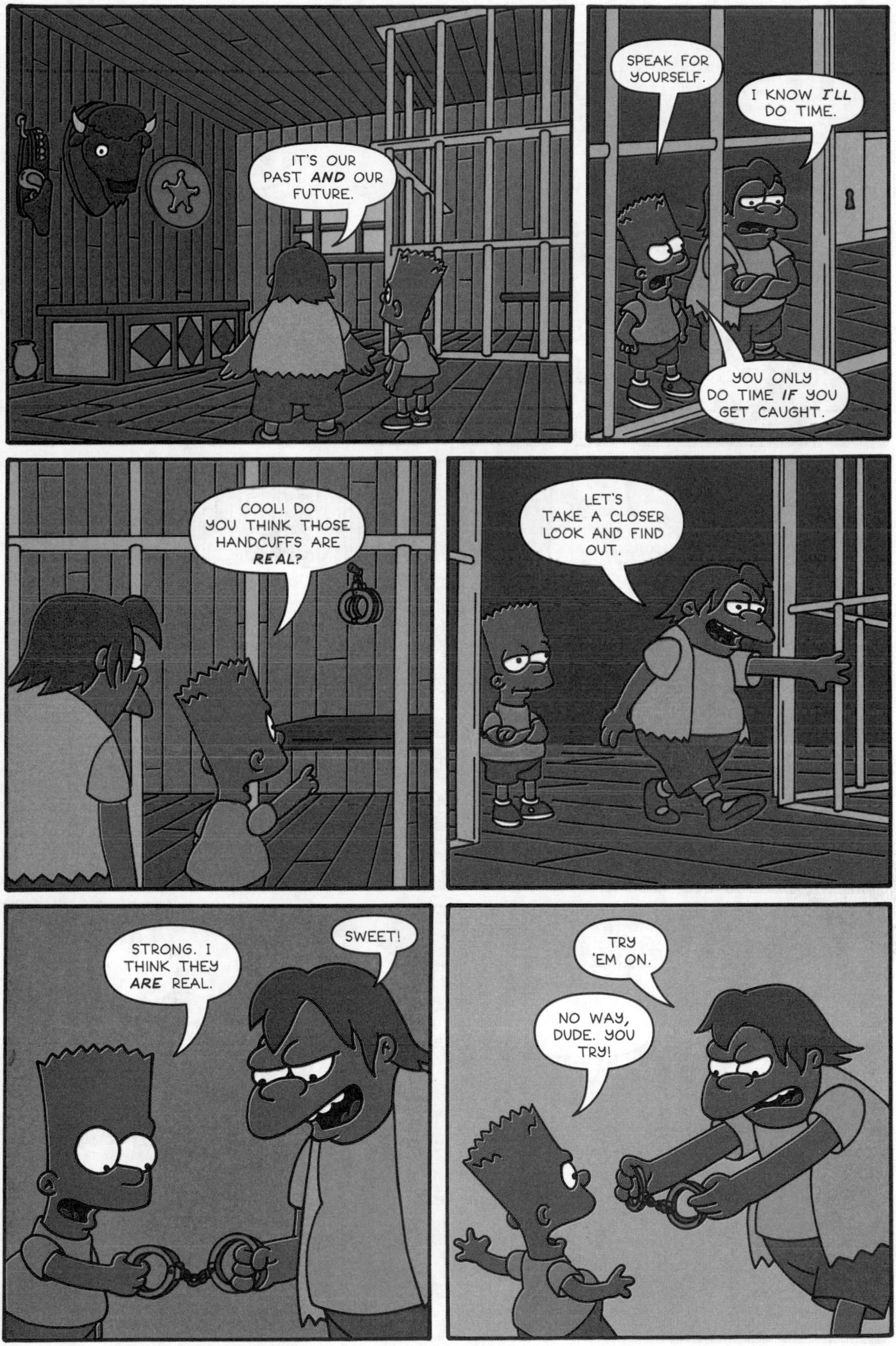
IT'S OUR PAST AND OUR FUTURE.
SPEAK FOR YOURSELF.
I KNOW I'LL DO TIME.
YOU ONLY DO TIME IF YOU GET CAUGHT.
COOL! DO YOU THINK THOSE HANDCUFFS ARE REAL?
LET'S TAKE A CLOSER LOOK AND FIND OUT.
STRONG. I THINK THEY ARE REAL.
SWEET!
TRY 'EM ON.
NO WAY, DUDE. YOU TRY!

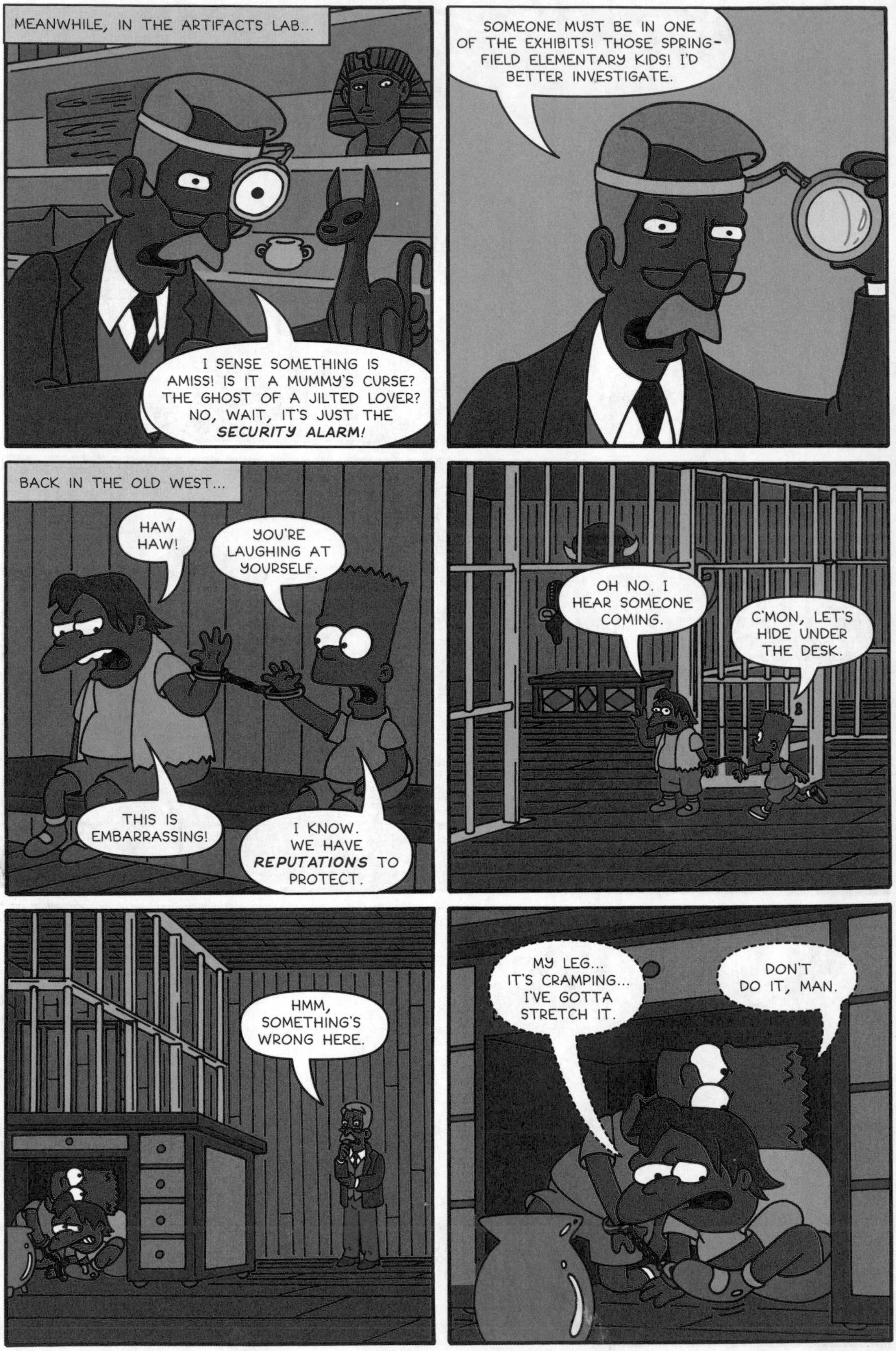
MEANWHILE, IN THE ARTIFACTS LAB...
I SENSE SOMETHING IS AMISS! IS IT A MUMMY'S CURSE? THE GHOST OF A JILTED LOVER? NO, WAIT, IT'S JUST THE **SECURITY ALARM!**
SOMEONE MUST BE IN ONE OF THE EXHIBITS! THOSE SPRING-FIELD ELEMENTARY KIDS! I'D BETTER INVESTIGATE.
BACK IN THE OLD WEST...
HAW HAW!
YOU'RE LAUGHING AT YOURSELF.
THIS IS EMBARRASSING!
I KNOW. WE HAVE **REPUTATIONS** TO PROTECT.
OH NO. I HEAR SOMEONE COMING.
C'MON, LET'S HIDE UNDER THE DESK.
HMM, SOMETHING'S WRONG HERE.
MY LEG... IT'S CRAMPING... I'VE GOTTA STRETCH IT.
DON'T DO IT, MAN.

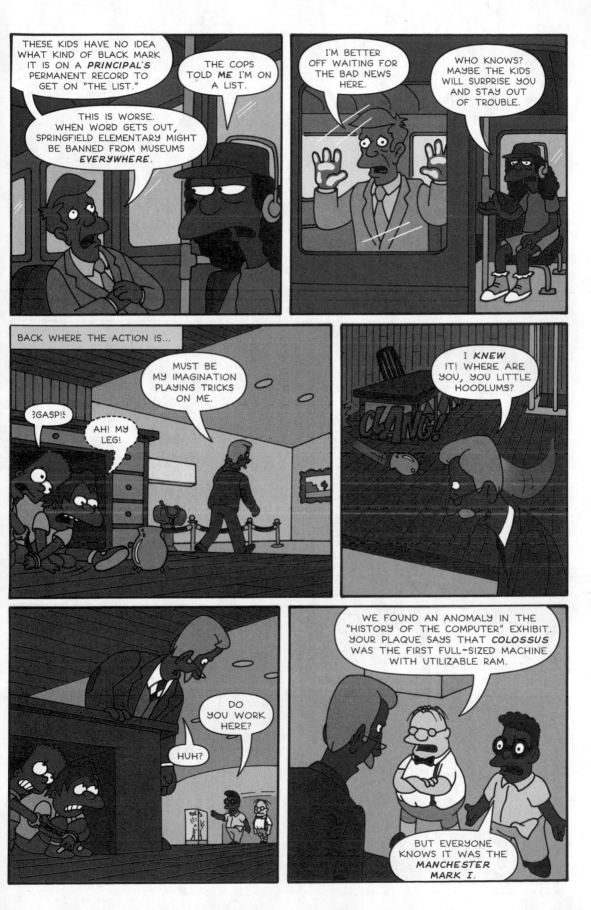

THESE KIDS HAVE NO IDEA WHAT KIND OF BLACK MARK IT IS ON A *PRINCIPAL'S* PERMANENT RECORD TO GET ON "THE LIST."

THE COPS TOLD *ME* I'M ON A LIST.

THIS IS WORSE. WHEN WORD GETS OUT, SPRINGFIELD ELEMENTARY MIGHT BE BANNED FROM MUSEUMS *EVERYWHERE*.

I'M BETTER OFF WAITING FOR THE BAD NEWS HERE.

WHO KNOWS? MAYBE THE KIDS WILL SURPRISE YOU AND STAY OUT OF TROUBLE.

BACK WHERE THE ACTION IS...

MUST BE MY IMAGINATION PLAYING TRICKS ON ME.

¡GASP!¡

AH! MY LEG!

CLANG!

I *KNEW* IT! WHERE ARE YOU, YOU LITTLE HOODLUMS?

DO YOU WORK HERE?

HUH?

WE FOUND AN ANOMALY IN THE "HISTORY OF THE COMPUTER" EXHIBIT. YOUR PLAQUE SAYS THAT *COLOSSUS* WAS THE FIRST FULL-SIZED MACHINE WITH UTILIZABLE RAM.

BUT EVERYONE KNOWS IT WAS THE *MANCHESTER MARK I*.

29

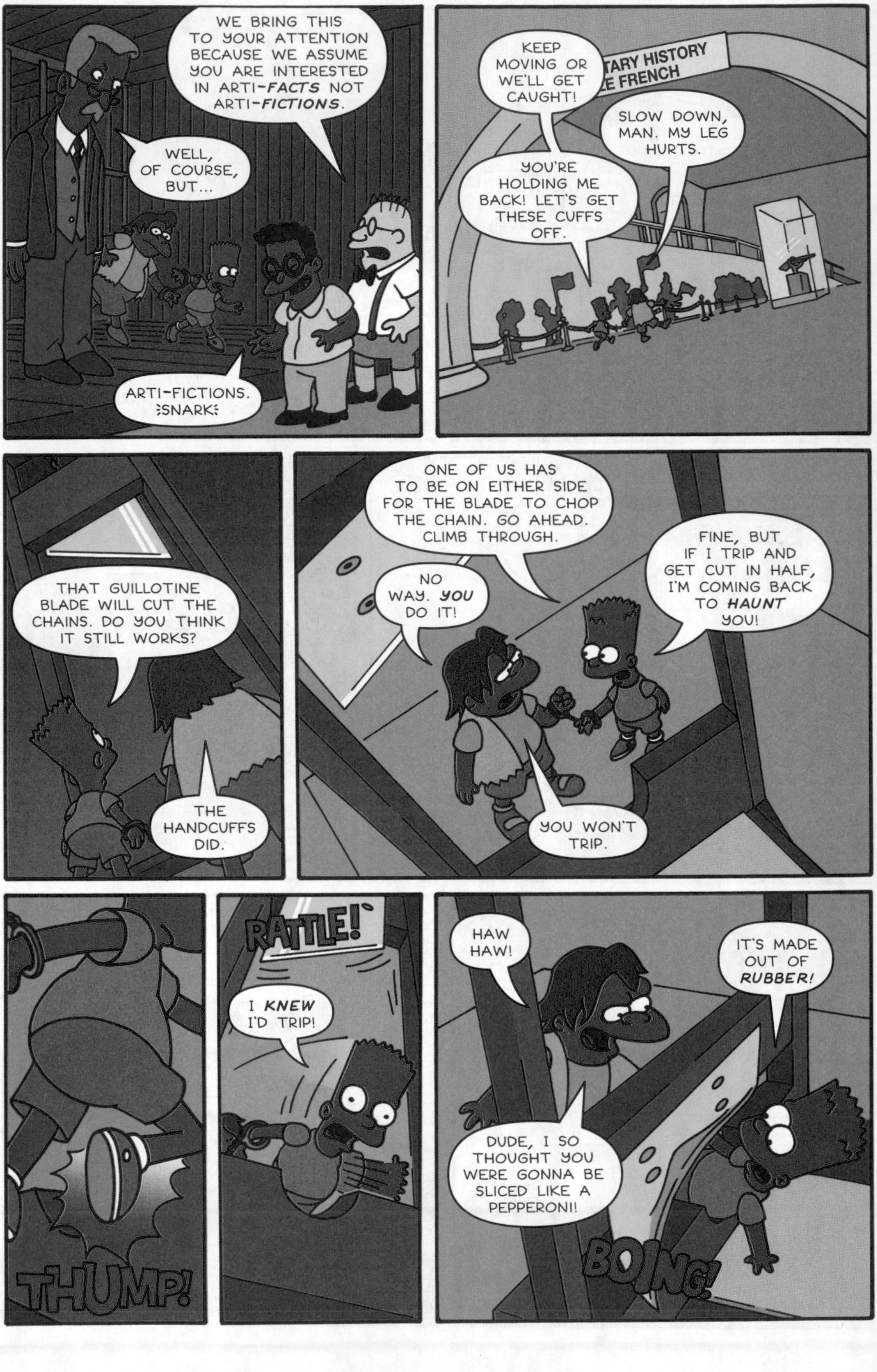
WE BRING THIS TO YOUR ATTENTION BECAUSE WE ASSUME YOU ARE INTERESTED IN ARTI-*FACTS* NOT ARTI-*FICTIONS*.
WELL, OF COURSE, BUT...
ARTI-FICTIONS. ›SNARK‹
KEEP MOVING OR WE'LL GET CAUGHT!
TARY HISTORY
E FRENCH
SLOW DOWN, MAN. MY LEG HURTS.
YOU'RE HOLDING ME BACK! LET'S GET THESE CUFFS OFF.
THAT GUILLOTINE BLADE WILL CUT THE CHAINS. DO YOU THINK IT STILL WORKS?
THE HANDCUFFS DID.
ONE OF US HAS TO BE ON EITHER SIDE FOR THE BLADE TO CHOP THE CHAIN. GO AHEAD. CLIMB THROUGH.
NO WAY. *YOU* DO IT!
FINE, BUT IF I TRIP AND GET CUT IN HALF, I'M COMING BACK TO *HAUNT* YOU!
YOU WON'T TRIP.
THUMP!
RATTLE!
I *KNEW* I'D TRIP!
HAW HAW!
IT'S MADE OUT OF *RUBBER!*
DUDE, I SO THOUGHT YOU WERE GONNA BE SLICED LIKE A PEPPERONI!
BOING!

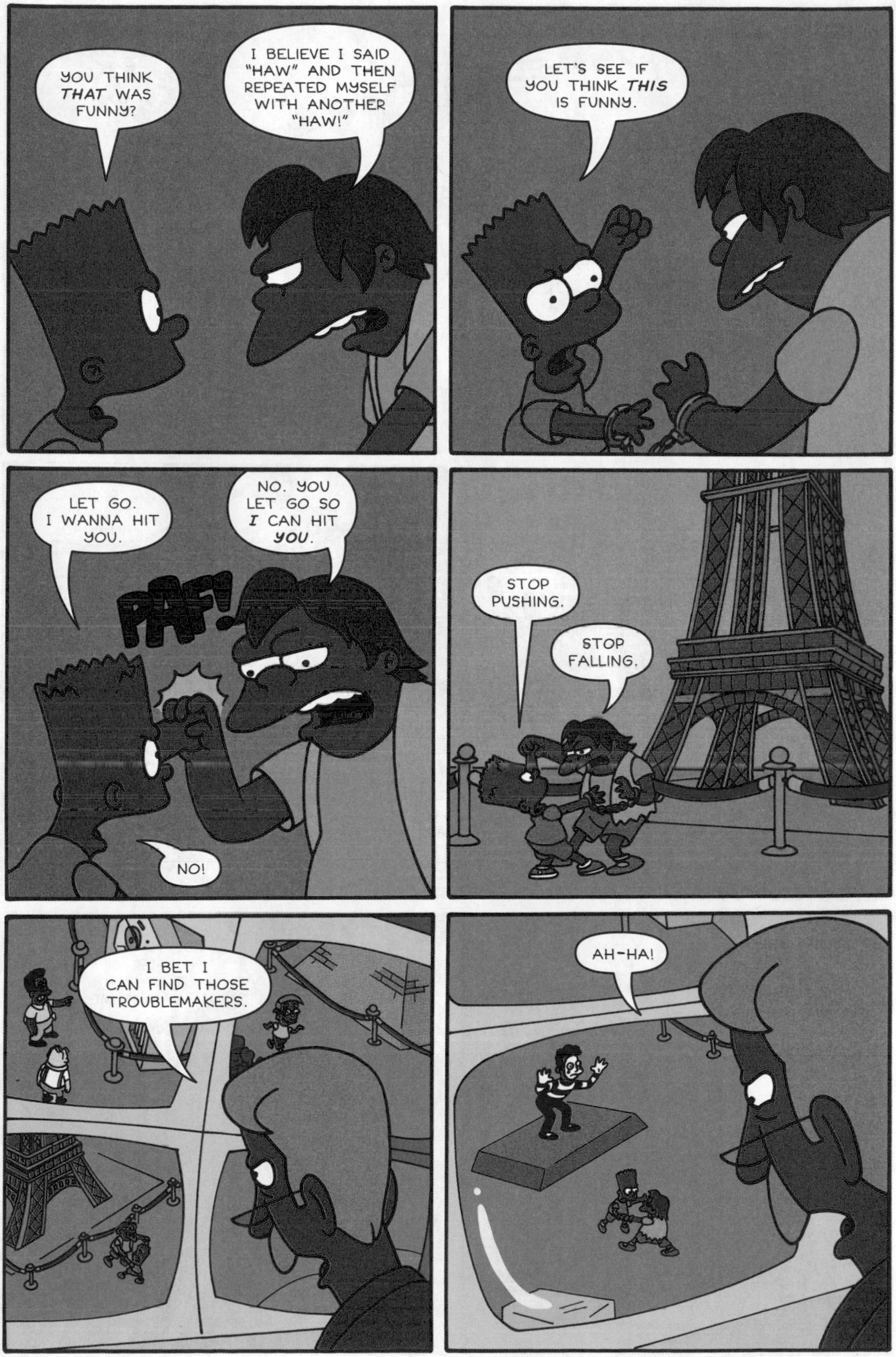
YOU THINK THAT WAS FUNNY?
I BELIEVE I SAID "HAW" AND THEN REPEATED MYSELF WITH ANOTHER "HAW!"
LET'S SEE IF YOU THINK THIS IS FUNNY.
LET GO. I WANNA HIT YOU.
NO. YOU LET GO SO I CAN HIT YOU.
PAF!
NO!
STOP PUSHING.
STOP FALLING.
I BET I CAN FIND THOSE TROUBLEMAKERS.
AH-HA!

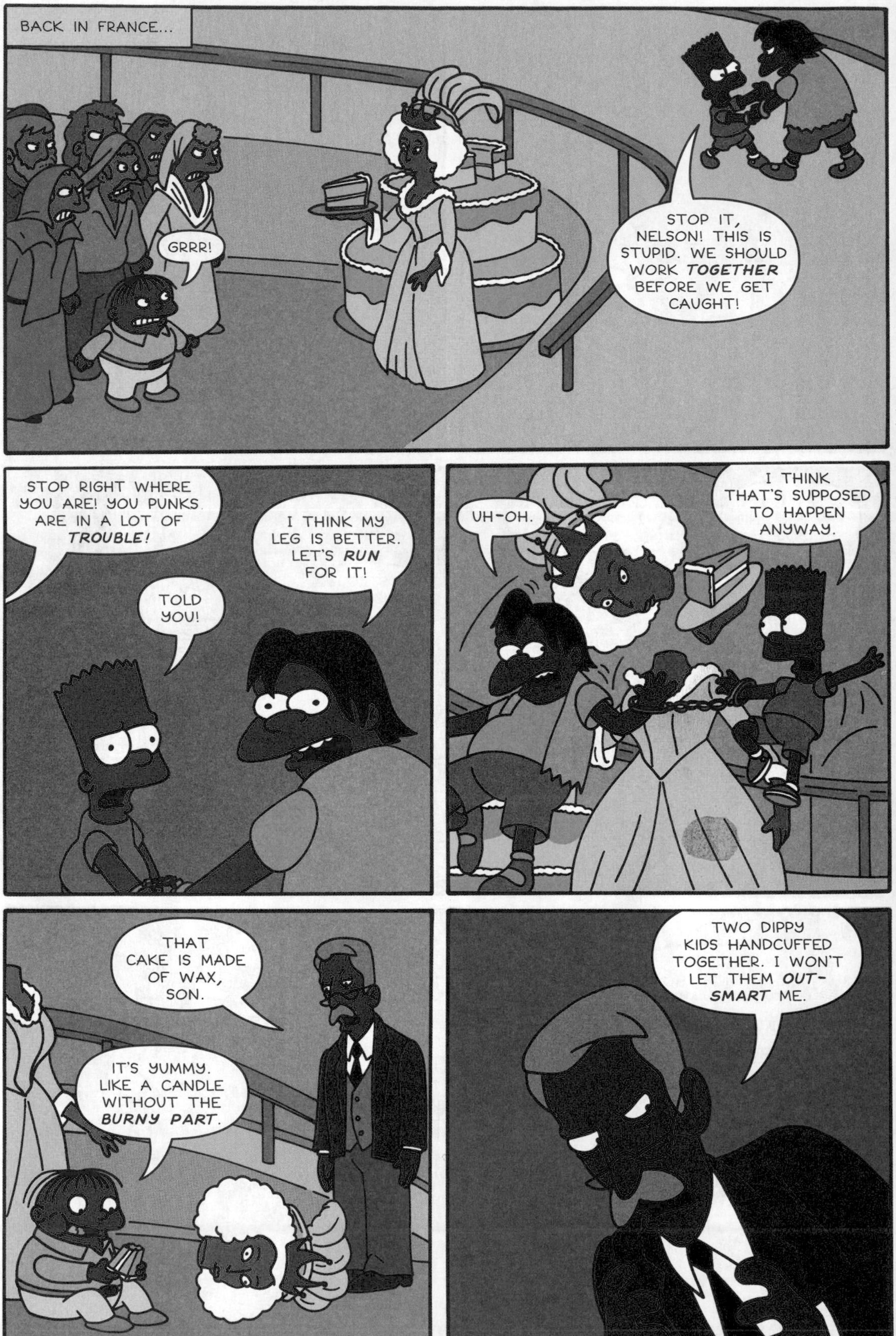
BACK IN FRANCE...
GRRR!
STOP IT, NELSON! THIS IS STUPID. WE SHOULD WORK *TOGETHER* BEFORE WE GET CAUGHT!
STOP RIGHT WHERE YOU ARE! YOU PUNKS ARE IN A LOT OF *TROUBLE!*
TOLD YOU!
I THINK MY LEG IS BETTER. LET'S *RUN* FOR IT!
UH-OH.
I THINK THAT'S SUPPOSED TO HAPPEN ANYWAY.
THAT CAKE IS MADE OF WAX, SON.
IT'S YUMMY. LIKE A CANDLE WITHOUT THE *BURNY PART*.
TWO DIPPY KIDS HANDCUFFED TOGETHER. I WON'T LET THEM *OUT-SMART* ME.

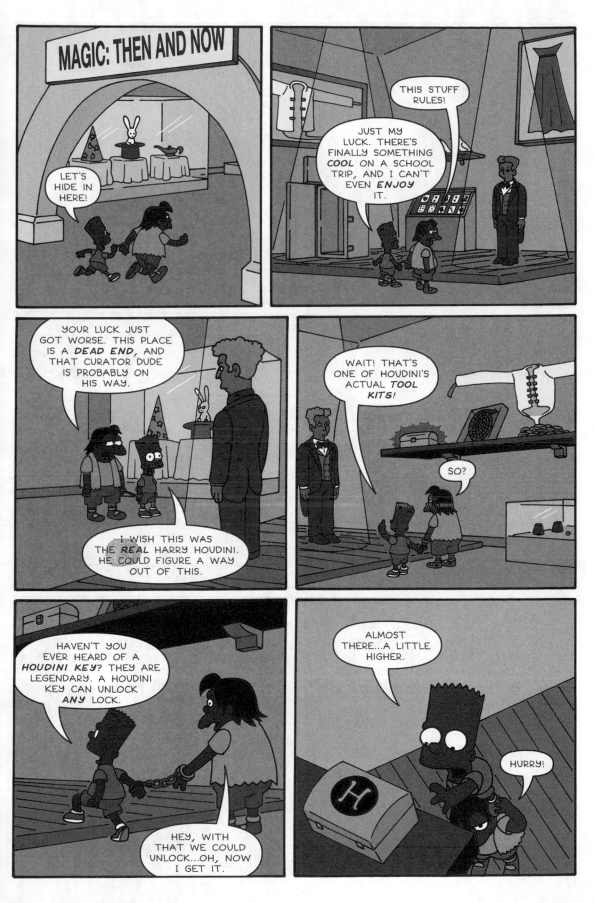

MAGIC: THEN AND NOW

LET'S HIDE IN HERE!

THIS STUFF RULES!

JUST MY LUCK. THERE'S FINALLY SOMETHING *COOL* ON A SCHOOL TRIP, AND I CAN'T EVEN *ENJOY* IT.

YOUR LUCK JUST GOT WORSE. THIS PLACE IS A *DEAD END,* AND THAT CURATOR DUDE IS PROBABLY ON HIS WAY.

I WISH THIS WAS THE *REAL* HARRY HOUDINI. HE COULD FIGURE A WAY OUT OF THIS.

WAIT! THAT'S ONE OF HOUDINI'S ACTUAL *TOOL KITS!*

SO?

HAVEN'T YOU EVER HEARD OF A *HOUDINI KEY?* THEY ARE LEGENDARY. A HOUDINI KEY CAN UNLOCK *ANY* LOCK.

HEY, WITH THAT WE COULD UNLOCK...OH, NOW I GET IT.

ALMOST THERE...A LITTLE HIGHER.

HURRY!

33

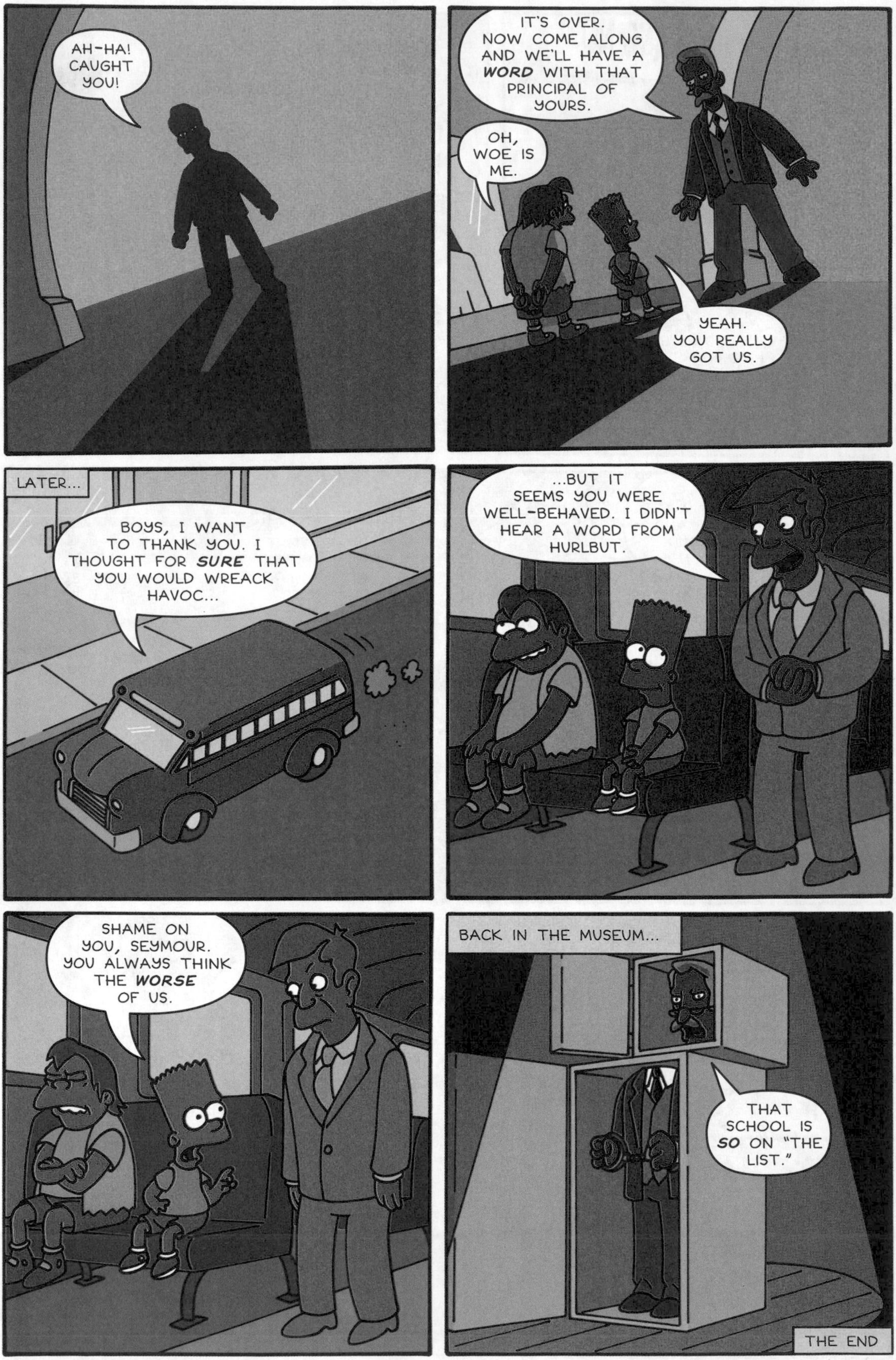
AH-HA! CAUGHT YOU!
IT'S OVER. NOW COME ALONG AND WE'LL HAVE A WORD WITH THAT PRINCIPAL OF YOURS.
OH, WOE IS ME.
YEAH. YOU REALLY GOT US.
LATER...
BOYS, I WANT TO THANK YOU. I THOUGHT FOR SURE THAT YOU WOULD WREACK HAVOC...
...BUT IT SEEMS YOU WERE WELL-BEHAVED. I DIDN'T HEAR A WORD FROM HURLBUT.
SHAME ON YOU, SEYMOUR. YOU ALWAYS THINK THE WORSE OF US.
BACK IN THE MUSEUM...
THAT SCHOOL IS SO ON "THE LIST."
THE END

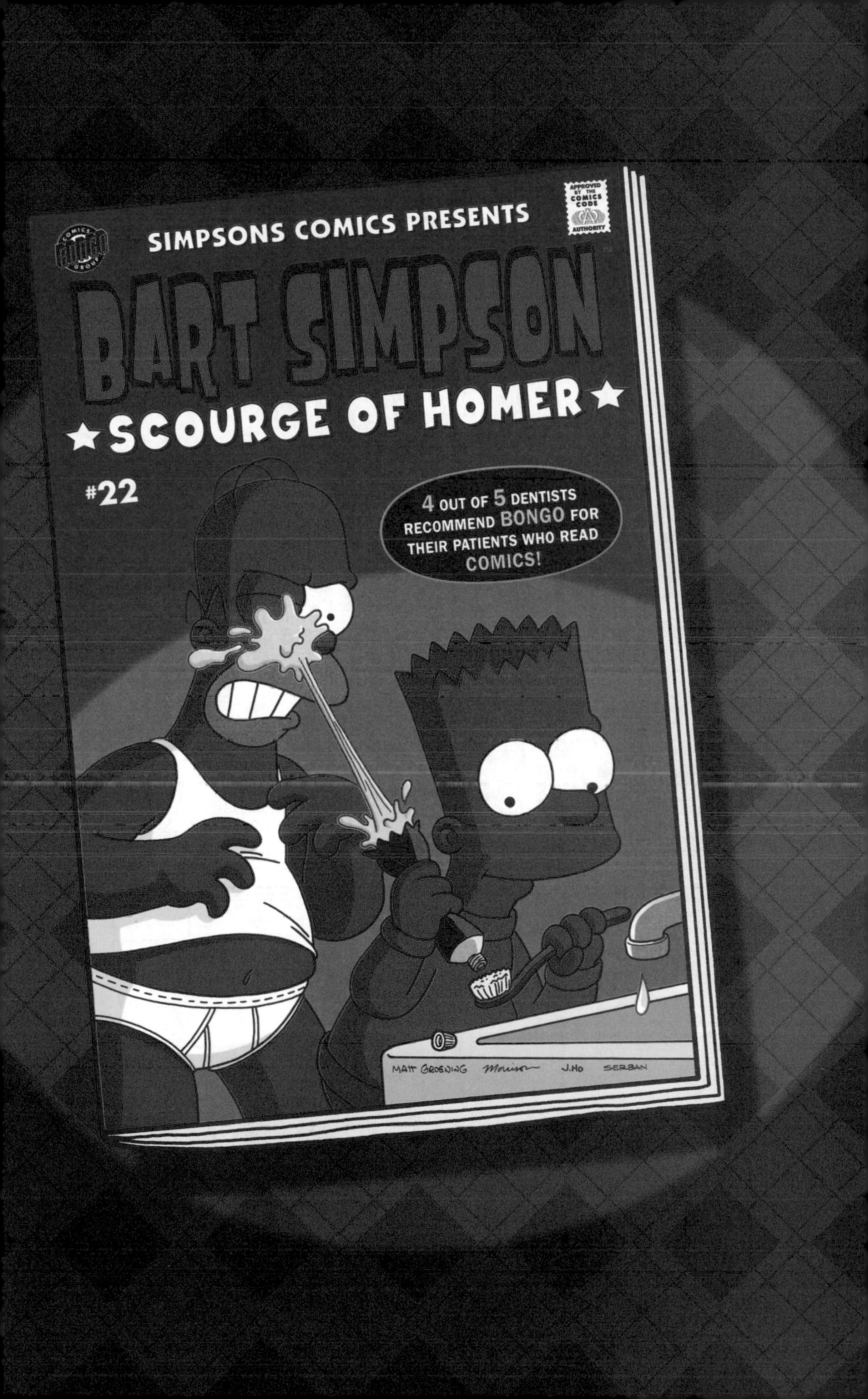
SIMPSONS COMICS PRESENTS
APPROVED BY THE COMICS CODE AUTHORITY
BART SIMPSON
★SCOURGE OF HOMER★
#22
4 OUT OF 5 DENTISTS RECOMMEND BONGO FOR THEIR PATIENTS WHO READ COMICS!
MATT GROENING
J.HO
SERBAN

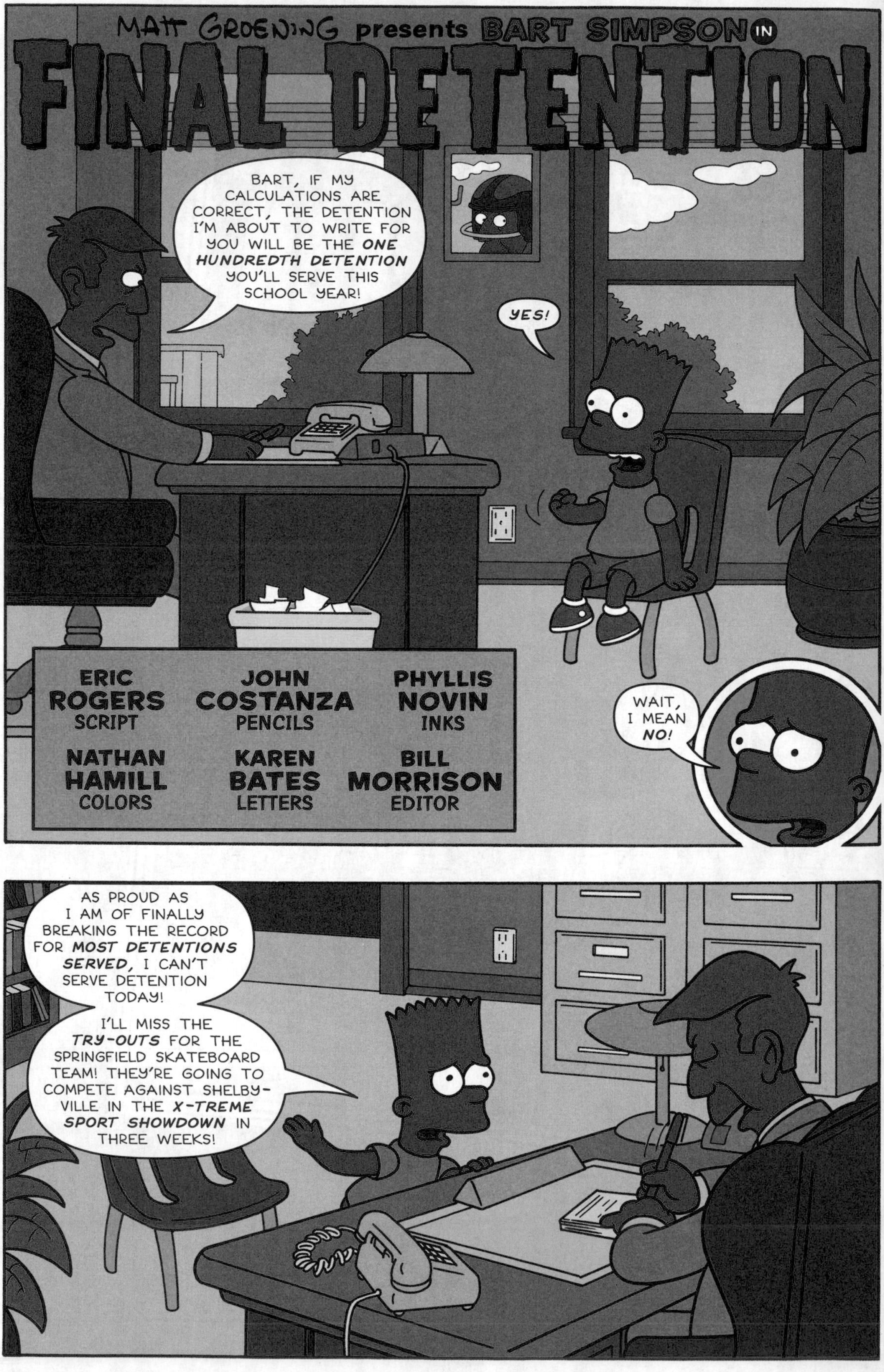

MATT GROENING presents BART SIMPSON IN
FINAL DETENTION
BART, IF MY CALCULATIONS ARE CORRECT, THE DETENTION I'M ABOUT TO WRITE FOR YOU WILL BE THE ONE HUNDREDTH DETENTION YOU'LL SERVE THIS SCHOOL YEAR!
YES!
ERIC ROGERS SCRIPT
JOHN COSTANZA PENCILS
PHYLLIS NOVIN INKS
NATHAN HAMILL COLORS
KAREN BATES LETTERS
BILL MORRISON EDITOR
WAIT, I MEAN NO!
AS PROUD AS I AM OF FINALLY BREAKING THE RECORD FOR MOST DETENTIONS SERVED, I CAN'T SERVE DETENTION TODAY!
I'LL MISS THE TRY-OUTS FOR THE SPRINGFIELD SKATEBOARD TEAM! THEY'RE GOING TO COMPETE AGAINST SHELBY-VILLE IN THE X-TREME SPORT SHOWDOWN IN THREE WEEKS!

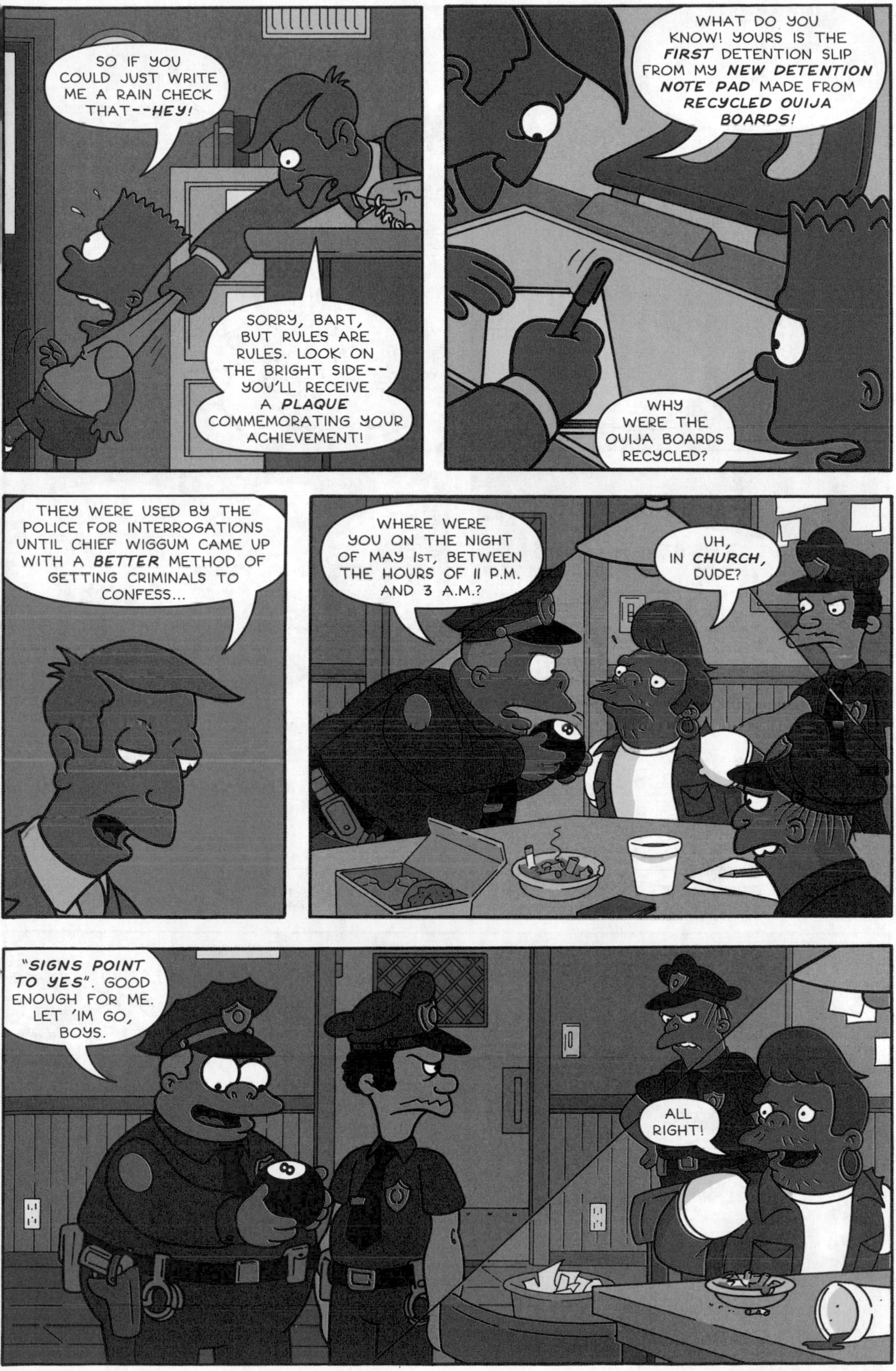
SO IF YOU COULD JUST WRITE ME A RAIN CHECK THAT--HEY!
SORRY, BART, BUT RULES ARE RULES. LOOK ON THE BRIGHT SIDE-- YOU'LL RECEIVE A PLAQUE COMMEMORATING YOUR ACHIEVEMENT!
WHAT DO YOU KNOW! YOURS IS THE FIRST DETENTION SLIP FROM MY NEW DETENTION NOTE PAD MADE FROM RECYCLED OUIJA BOARDS!
WHY WERE THE OUIJA BOARDS RECYCLED?
THEY WERE USED BY THE POLICE FOR INTERROGATIONS UNTIL CHIEF WIGGUM CAME UP WITH A BETTER METHOD OF GETTING CRIMINALS TO CONFESS...
WHERE WERE YOU ON THE NIGHT OF MAY 1st, BETWEEN THE HOURS OF 11 P.M. AND 3 A.M.?
UH, IN CHURCH, DUDE?
8
"SIGNS POINT TO YES". GOOD ENOUGH FOR ME. LET 'IM GO, BOYS.
8
ALL RIGHT!

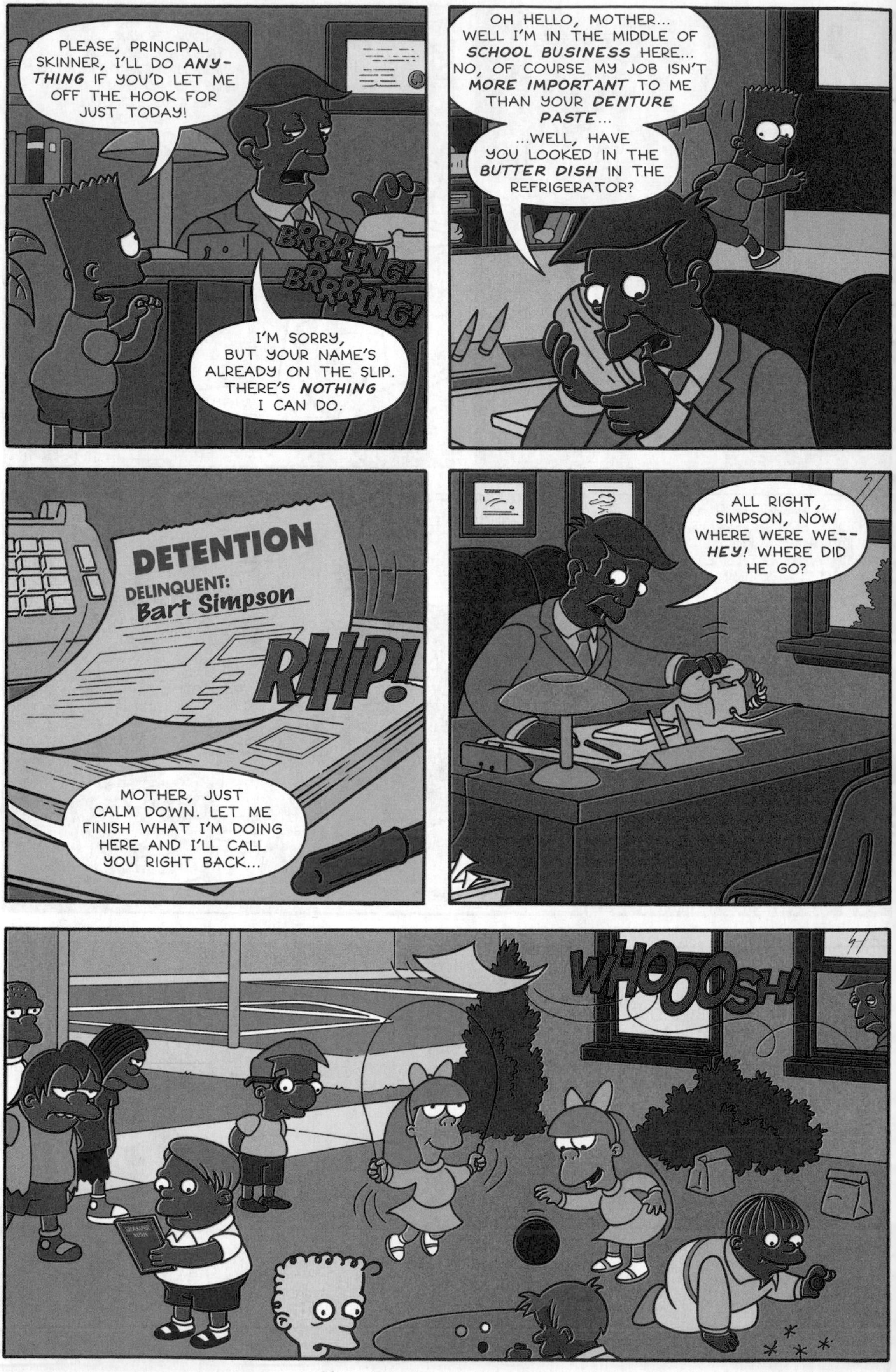
PLEASE, PRINCIPAL SKINNER, I'LL DO ANY-THING IF YOU'D LET ME OFF THE HOOK FOR JUST TODAY!
BRRRING! BRRRING!
I'M SORRY, BUT YOUR NAME'S ALREADY ON THE SLIP. THERE'S NOTHING I CAN DO.
OH HELLO, MOTHER... WELL I'M IN THE MIDDLE OF SCHOOL BUSINESS HERE... NO, OF COURSE MY JOB ISN'T MORE IMPORTANT TO ME THAN YOUR DENTURE PASTE...
...WELL, HAVE YOU LOOKED IN THE BUTTER DISH IN THE REFRIGERATOR?
DETENTION
DELINQUENT:
Bart Simpson
RIIIP!
MOTHER, JUST CALM DOWN. LET ME FINISH WHAT I'M DOING HERE AND I'LL CALL YOU RIGHT BACK...
ALL RIGHT, SIMPSON, NOW WHERE WERE WE-- HEY! WHERE DID HE GO?
WHOOOSH!

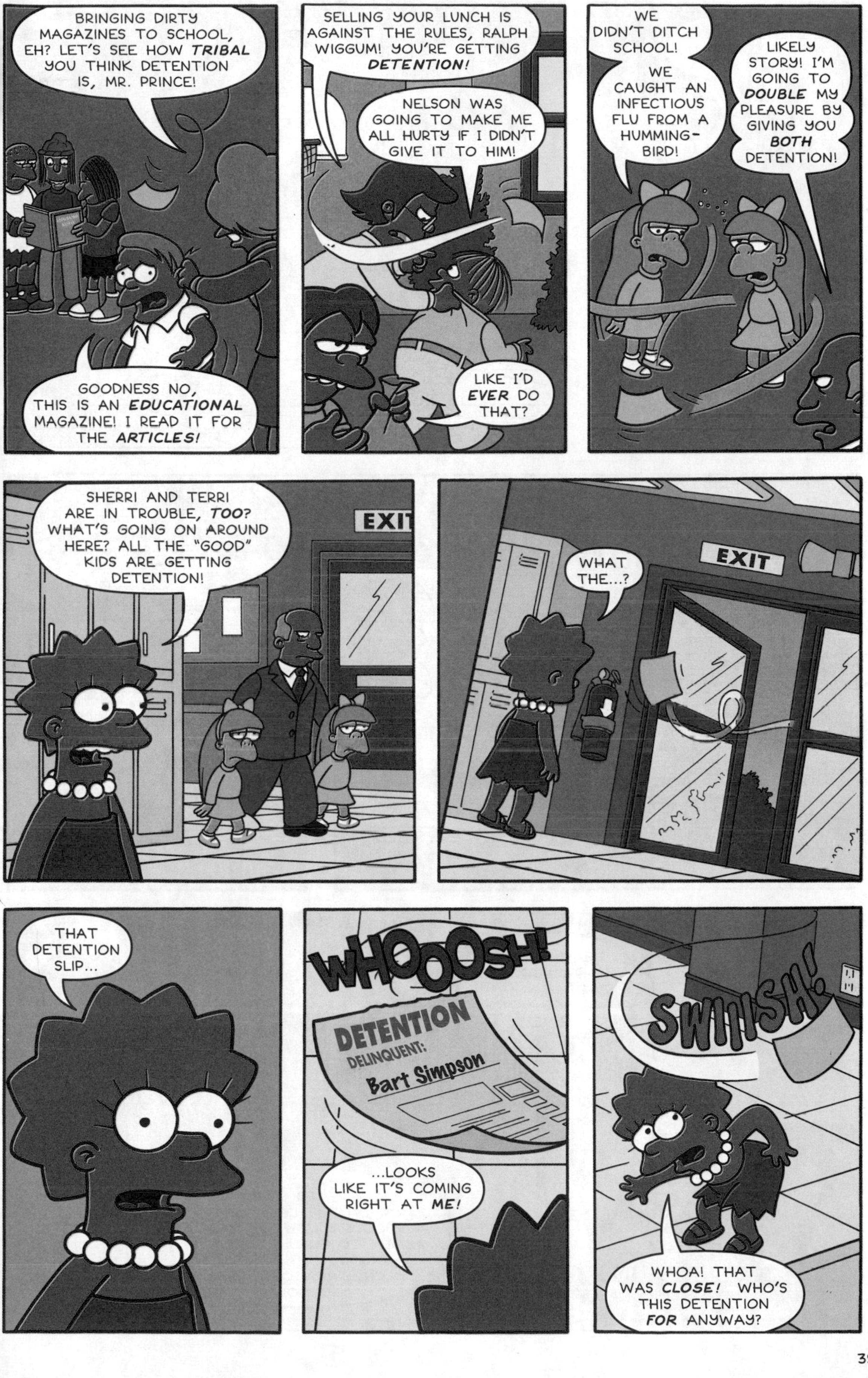
BRINGING DIRTY MAGAZINES TO SCHOOL, EH? LET'S SEE HOW *TRIBAL* YOU THINK DETENTION IS, MR. PRINCE!
GOODNESS NO, THIS IS AN *EDUCATIONAL* MAGAZINE! I READ IT FOR THE *ARTICLES!*
SELLING YOUR LUNCH IS AGAINST THE RULES, RALPH WIGGUM! YOU'RE GETTING *DETENTION!*
NELSON WAS GOING TO MAKE ME ALL HURTY IF I DIDN'T GIVE IT TO HIM!
LIKE I'D *EVER* DO THAT?
WE DIDN'T DITCH SCHOOL!
WE CAUGHT AN INFECTIOUS FLU FROM A HUMMING-BIRD!
LIKELY STORY! I'M GOING TO *DOUBLE* MY PLEASURE BY GIVING YOU *BOTH* DETENTION!
SHERRI AND TERRI ARE IN TROUBLE, *TOO*? WHAT'S GOING ON AROUND HERE? ALL THE "GOOD" KIDS ARE GETTING DETENTION!
EXIT
WHAT THE...?
EXIT
THAT DETENTION SLIP...
WHOOOSH!
DETENTION
DELINQUENT:
Bart Simpson
...LOOKS LIKE IT'S COMING RIGHT AT *ME!*
SWIIISH!
WHOA! THAT WAS *CLOSE!* WHO'S THIS DETENTION *FOR* ANYWAY?

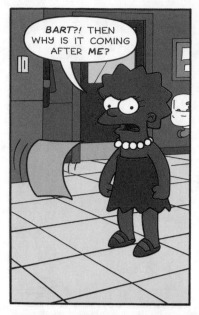

BART?! THEN WHY IS IT COMING AFTER *ME?*

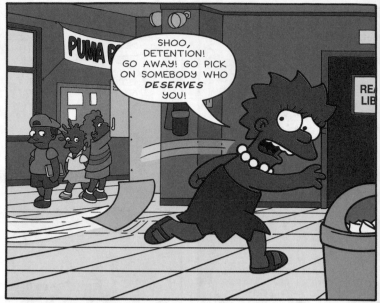

SHOO, DETENTION! GO AWAY! GO PICK ON SOMEBODY WHO *DESERVES* YOU!

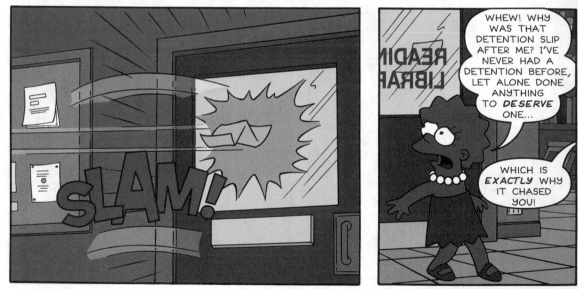

SLAM!

WHEW! WHY WAS THAT DETENTION SLIP AFTER ME? I'VE NEVER HAD A DETENTION BEFORE, LET ALONE DONE ANYTHING TO *DESERVE* ONE...

WHICH IS *EXACTLY* WHY IT CHASED YOU!

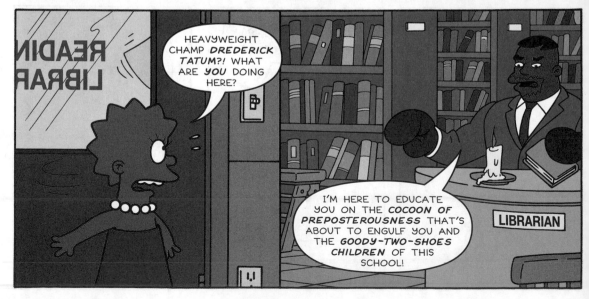

HEAVYWEIGHT CHAMP *DREDERICK TATUM?!* WHAT ARE *YOU* DOING HERE?

I'M HERE TO EDUCATE YOU ON THE *COCOON OF PREPOSTEROUSNESS* THAT'S ABOUT TO ENGULF YOU AND THE *GOODY-TWO-SHOES CHILDREN* OF THIS SCHOOL!

LIBRARIAN

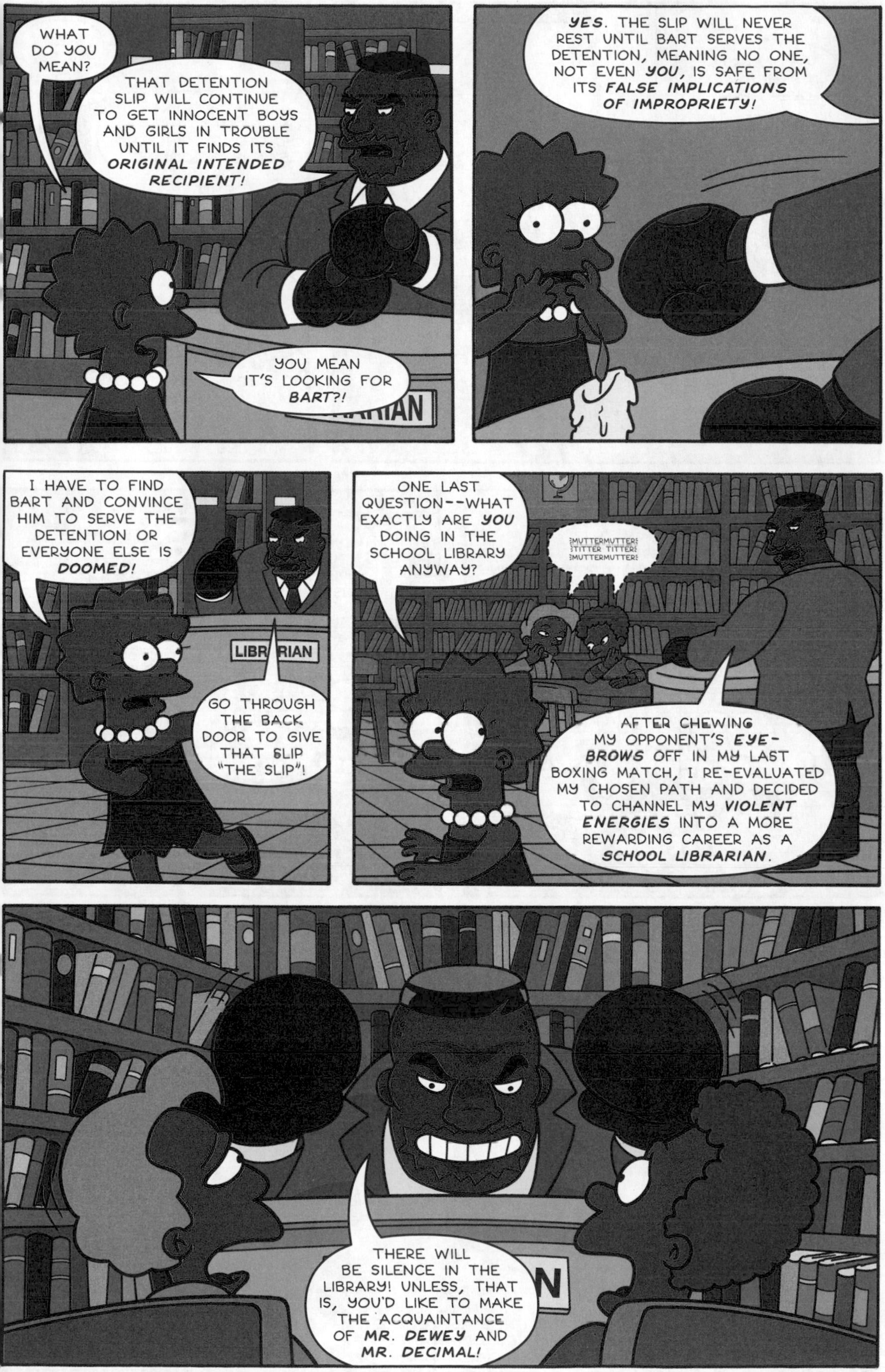
WHAT DO YOU MEAN?
THAT DETENTION SLIP WILL CONTINUE TO GET INNOCENT BOYS AND GIRLS IN TROUBLE UNTIL IT FINDS ITS ORIGINAL INTENDED RECIPIENT!
YOU MEAN IT'S LOOKING FOR BART?!
YES. THE SLIP WILL NEVER REST UNTIL BART SERVES THE DETENTION, MEANING NO ONE, NOT EVEN YOU, IS SAFE FROM ITS FALSE IMPLICATIONS OF IMPROPRIETY!
I HAVE TO FIND BART AND CONVINCE HIM TO SERVE THE DETENTION OR EVERYONE ELSE IS DOOMED!
LIBRARIAN
GO THROUGH THE BACK DOOR TO GIVE THAT SLIP "THE SLIP"!
ONE LAST QUESTION--WHAT EXACTLY ARE YOU DOING IN THE SCHOOL LIBRARY ANYWAY?
MUTTERMUTTER TITTER TITTER MUTTERMUTTER
AFTER CHEWING MY OPPONENT'S EYE-BROWS OFF IN MY LAST BOXING MATCH, I RE-EVALUATED MY CHOSEN PATH AND DECIDED TO CHANNEL MY VIOLENT ENERGIES INTO A MORE REWARDING CAREER AS A SCHOOL LIBRARIAN.
THERE WILL BE SILENCE IN THE LIBRARY! UNLESS, THAT IS, YOU'D LIKE TO MAKE THE ACQUAINTANCE OF MR. DEWEY AND MR. DECIMAL!

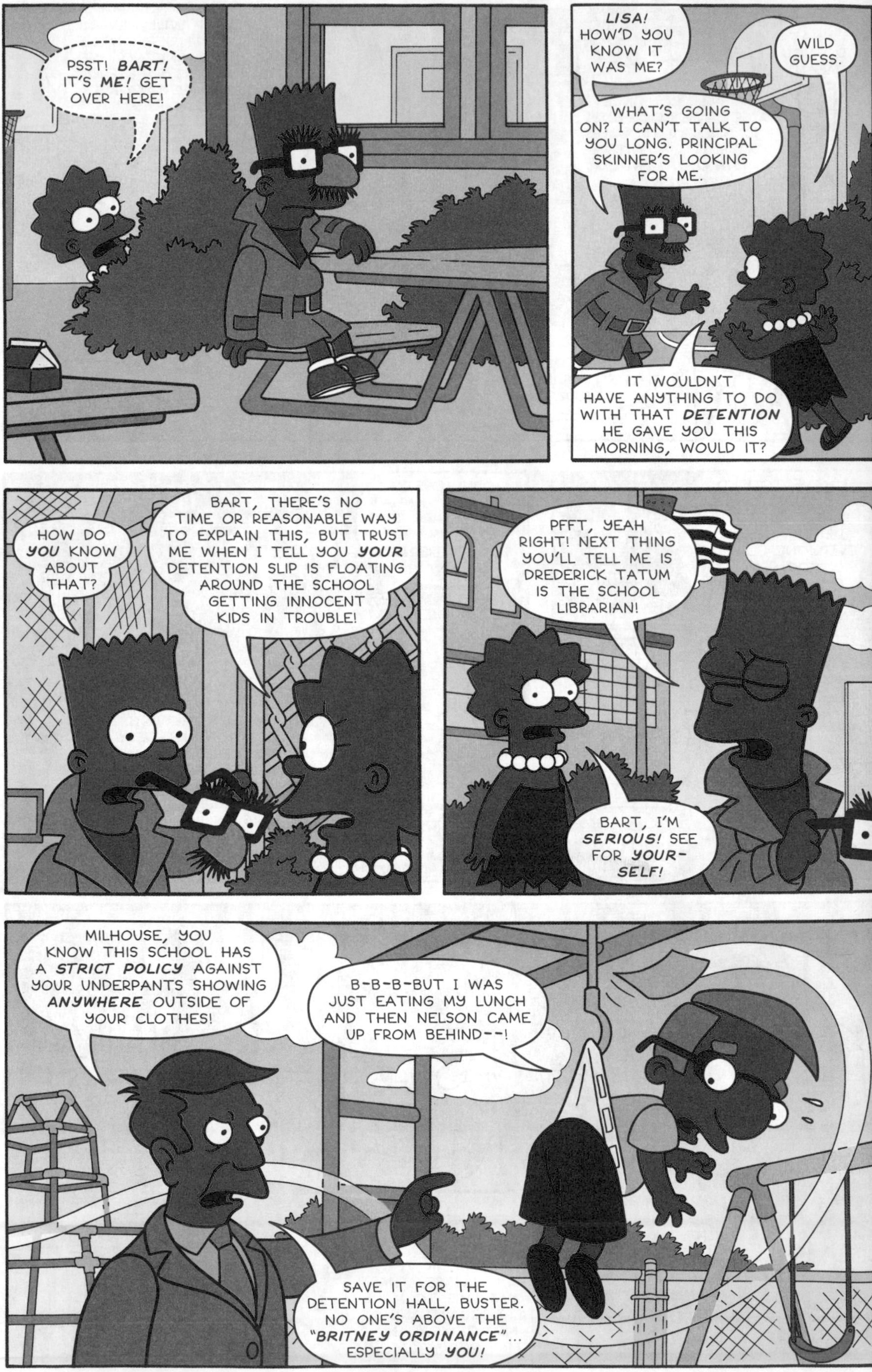
PSST! BART! IT'S ME! GET OVER HERE!
LISA! HOW'D YOU KNOW IT WAS ME?
WILD GUESS.
WHAT'S GOING ON? I CAN'T TALK TO YOU LONG. PRINCIPAL SKINNER'S LOOKING FOR ME.
IT WOULDN'T HAVE ANYTHING TO DO WITH THAT DETENTION HE GAVE YOU THIS MORNING, WOULD IT?
HOW DO YOU KNOW ABOUT THAT?
BART, THERE'S NO TIME OR REASONABLE WAY TO EXPLAIN THIS, BUT TRUST ME WHEN I TELL YOU YOUR DETENTION SLIP IS FLOATING AROUND THE SCHOOL GETTING INNOCENT KIDS IN TROUBLE!
PFFT, YEAH RIGHT! NEXT THING YOU'LL TELL ME IS DREDERICK TATUM IS THE SCHOOL LIBRARIAN!
BART, I'M SERIOUS! SEE FOR YOURSELF!
MILHOUSE, YOU KNOW THIS SCHOOL HAS A STRICT POLICY AGAINST YOUR UNDERPANTS SHOWING ANYWHERE OUTSIDE OF YOUR CLOTHES!
B-B-B-BUT I WAS JUST EATING MY LUNCH AND THEN NELSON CAME UP FROM BEHIND--!
SAVE IT FOR THE DETENTION HALL, BUSTER. NO ONE'S ABOVE THE "BRITNEY ORDINANCE"... ESPECIALLY YOU!

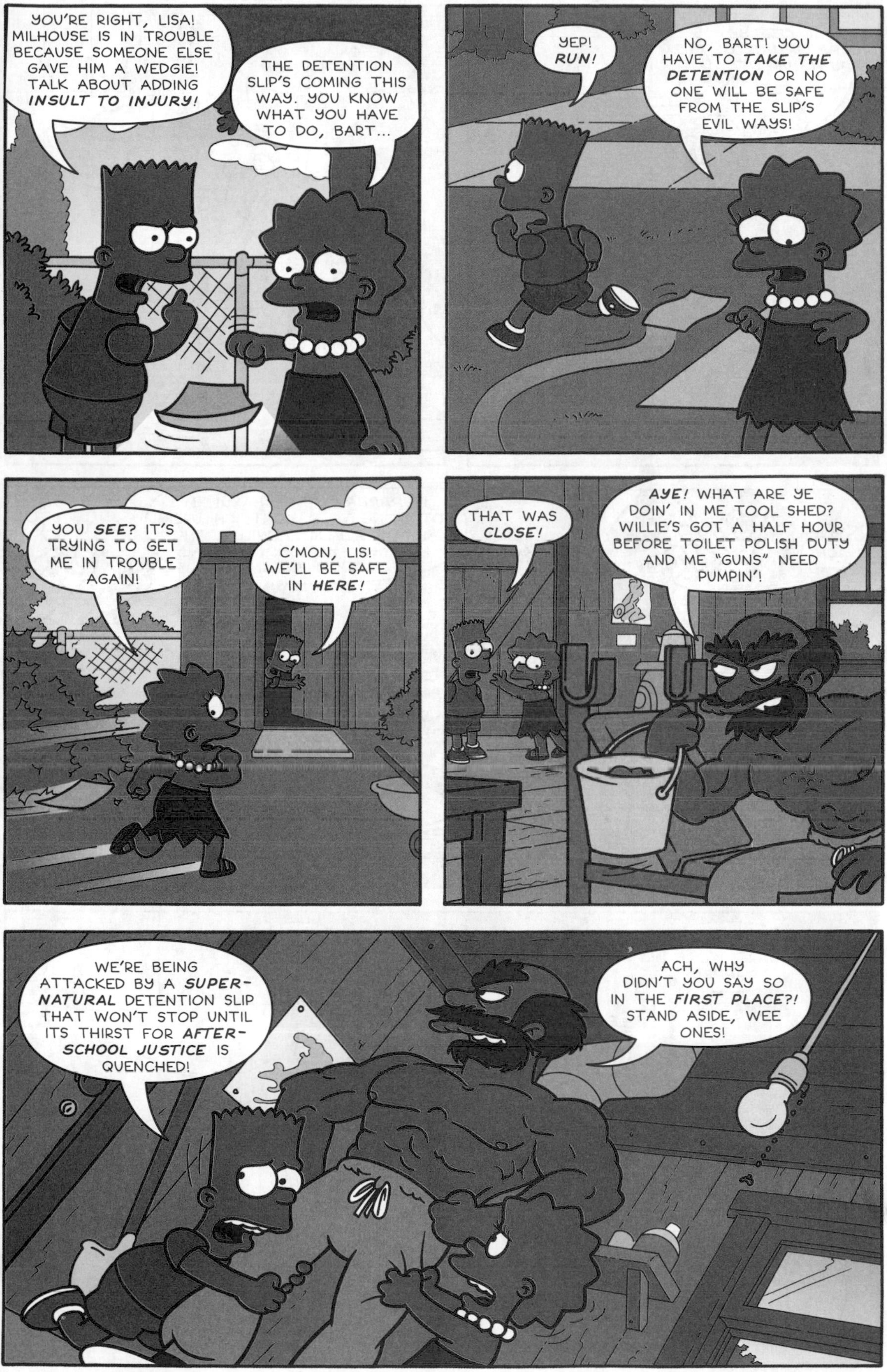
YOU'RE RIGHT, LISA! MILHOUSE IS IN TROUBLE BECAUSE SOMEONE ELSE GAVE HIM A WEDGIE! TALK ABOUT ADDING *INSULT TO INJURY*!
THE DETENTION SLIP'S COMING THIS WAY. YOU KNOW WHAT YOU HAVE TO DO, BART...
YEP! *RUN*!
NO, BART! YOU HAVE TO *TAKE THE DETENTION* OR NO ONE WILL BE SAFE FROM THE SLIP'S EVIL WAYS!
YOU *SEE*? IT'S TRYING TO GET ME IN TROUBLE AGAIN!
C'MON, LIS! WE'LL BE SAFE IN *HERE*!
THAT WAS *CLOSE*!
AYE! WHAT ARE YE DOIN' IN ME TOOL SHED? WILLIE'S GOT A HALF HOUR BEFORE TOILET POLISH DUTY AND ME "GUNS" NEED PUMPIN'!
WE'RE BEING ATTACKED BY A *SUPER-NATURAL* DETENTION SLIP THAT WON'T STOP UNTIL ITS THIRST FOR *AFTER-SCHOOL JUSTICE* IS QUENCHED!
ACH, WHY DIDN'T YOU SAY SO IN THE *FIRST PLACE*?! STAND ASIDE, WEE ONES!

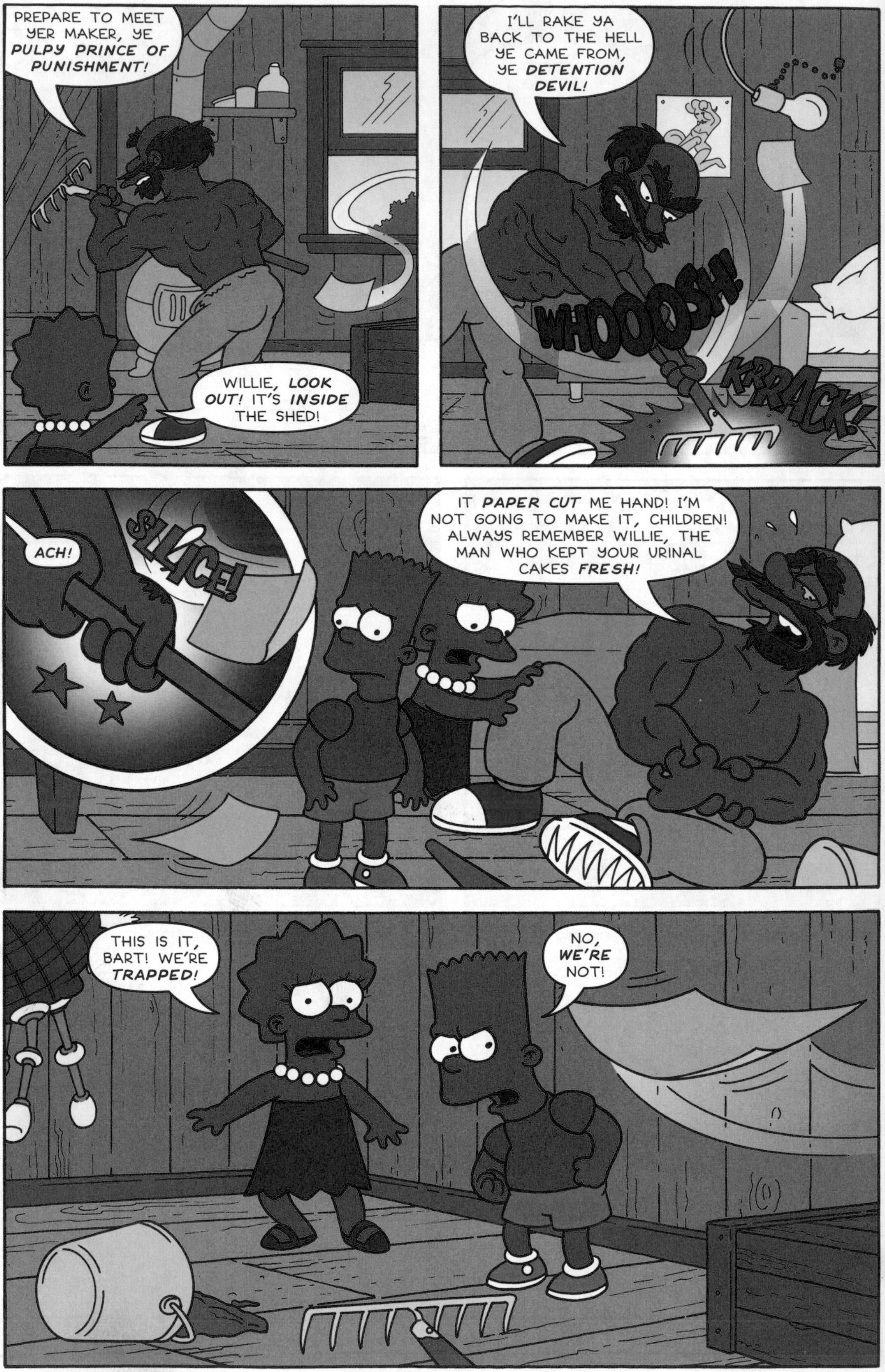
PREPARE TO MEET YER MAKER, YE PULPY PRINCE OF PUNISHMENT!
WILLIE, LOOK OUT! IT'S INSIDE THE SHED!
I'LL RAKE YA BACK TO THE HELL YE CAME FROM, YE DETENTION DEVIL!
WHOOOOSH!
KRRACK!
ACH!
SLLICE!
IT PAPER CUT ME HAND! I'M NOT GOING TO MAKE IT, CHILDREN! ALWAYS REMEMBER WILLIE, THE MAN WHO KEPT YOUR URINAL CAKES FRESH!
THIS IS IT, BART! WE'RE TRAPPED!
NO, WE'RE NOT!

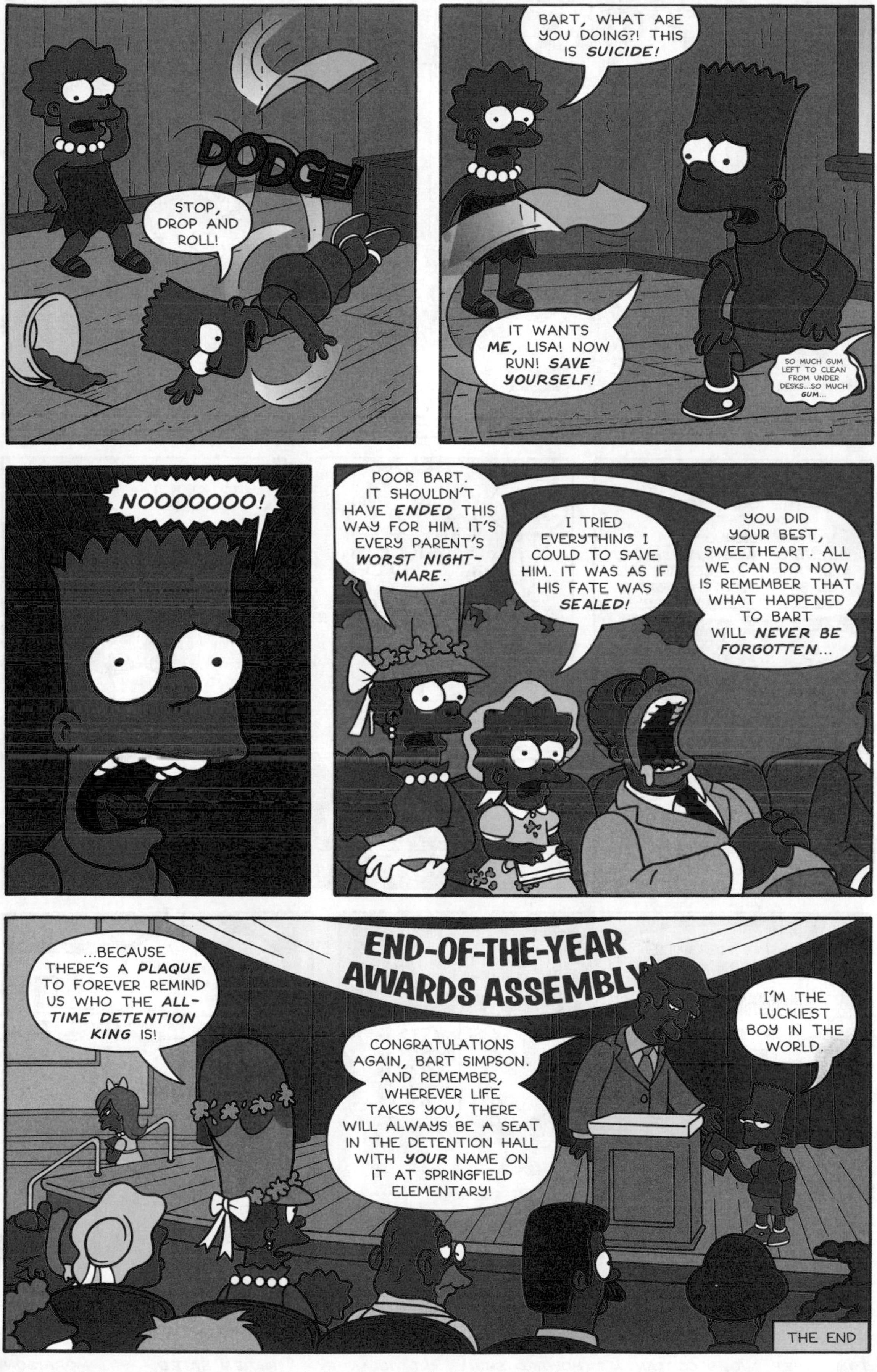
DODGE!
STOP, DROP AND ROLL!
BART, WHAT ARE YOU DOING?! THIS IS SUICIDE!
IT WANTS ME, LISA! NOW RUN! SAVE YOURSELF!
SO MUCH GUM LEFT TO CLEAN FROM UNDER DESKS...SO MUCH GUM...
NOOOOOOO!
POOR BART. IT SHOULDN'T HAVE ENDED THIS WAY FOR HIM. IT'S EVERY PARENT'S WORST NIGHT-MARE.
I TRIED EVERYTHING I COULD TO SAVE HIM. IT WAS AS IF HIS FATE WAS SEALED!
YOU DID YOUR BEST, SWEETHEART. ALL WE CAN DO NOW IS REMEMBER THAT WHAT HAPPENED TO BART WILL NEVER BE FORGOTTEN...
END-OF-THE-YEAR AWARDS ASSEMBLY
...BECAUSE THERE'S A PLAQUE TO FOREVER REMIND US WHO THE ALL-TIME DETENTION KING IS!
CONGRATULATIONS AGAIN, BART SIMPSON. AND REMEMBER, WHEREVER LIFE TAKES YOU, THERE WILL ALWAYS BE A SEAT IN THE DETENTION HALL WITH YOUR NAME ON IT AT SPRINGFIELD ELEMENTARY!
I'M THE LUCKIEST BOY IN THE WORLD.
THE END

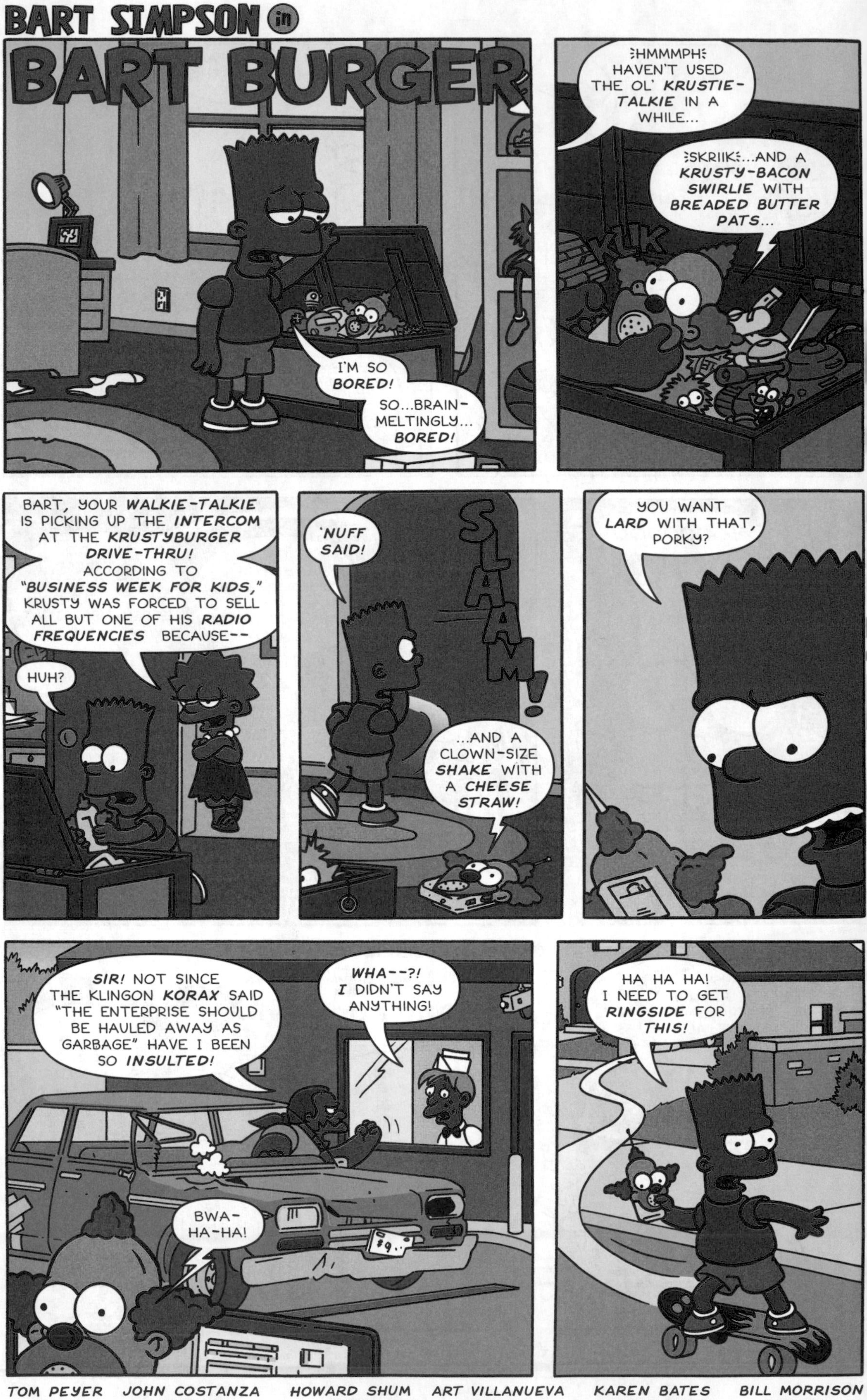
BART SIMPSON in
BART BURGER
I'M SO BORED!
SO...BRAIN-MELTINGLY... BORED!
HMMMPH HAVEN'T USED THE OL' KRUSTIE-TALKIE IN A WHILE...
KLIK
SKRIIK ...AND A KRUSTY-BACON SWIRLIE WITH BREADED BUTTER PATS...
BART, YOUR WALKIE-TALKIE IS PICKING UP THE INTERCOM AT THE KRUSTYBURGER DRIVE-THRU! ACCORDING TO "BUSINESS WEEK FOR KIDS," KRUSTY WAS FORCED TO SELL ALL BUT ONE OF HIS RADIO FREQUENCIES BECAUSE--
HUH?
'NUFF SAID!
SLAAAM!
...AND A CLOWN-SIZE SHAKE WITH A CHEESE STRAW!
YOU WANT LARD WITH THAT, PORKY?
SIR! NOT SINCE THE KLINGON KORAX SAID "THE ENTERPRISE SHOULD BE HAULED AWAY AS GARBAGE" HAVE I BEEN SO INSULTED!
WHA--?! I DIDN'T SAY ANYTHING!
BWA-HA-HA!
HA HA HA! I NEED TO GET RINGSIDE FOR THIS!

TOM PEYER SCRIPT · **JOHN COSTANZA** PENCILS · **HOWARD SHUM** INKS · **ART VILLANUEVA** COLORS · **KAREN BATES** LETTERS · **BILL MORRISON** EDITOR

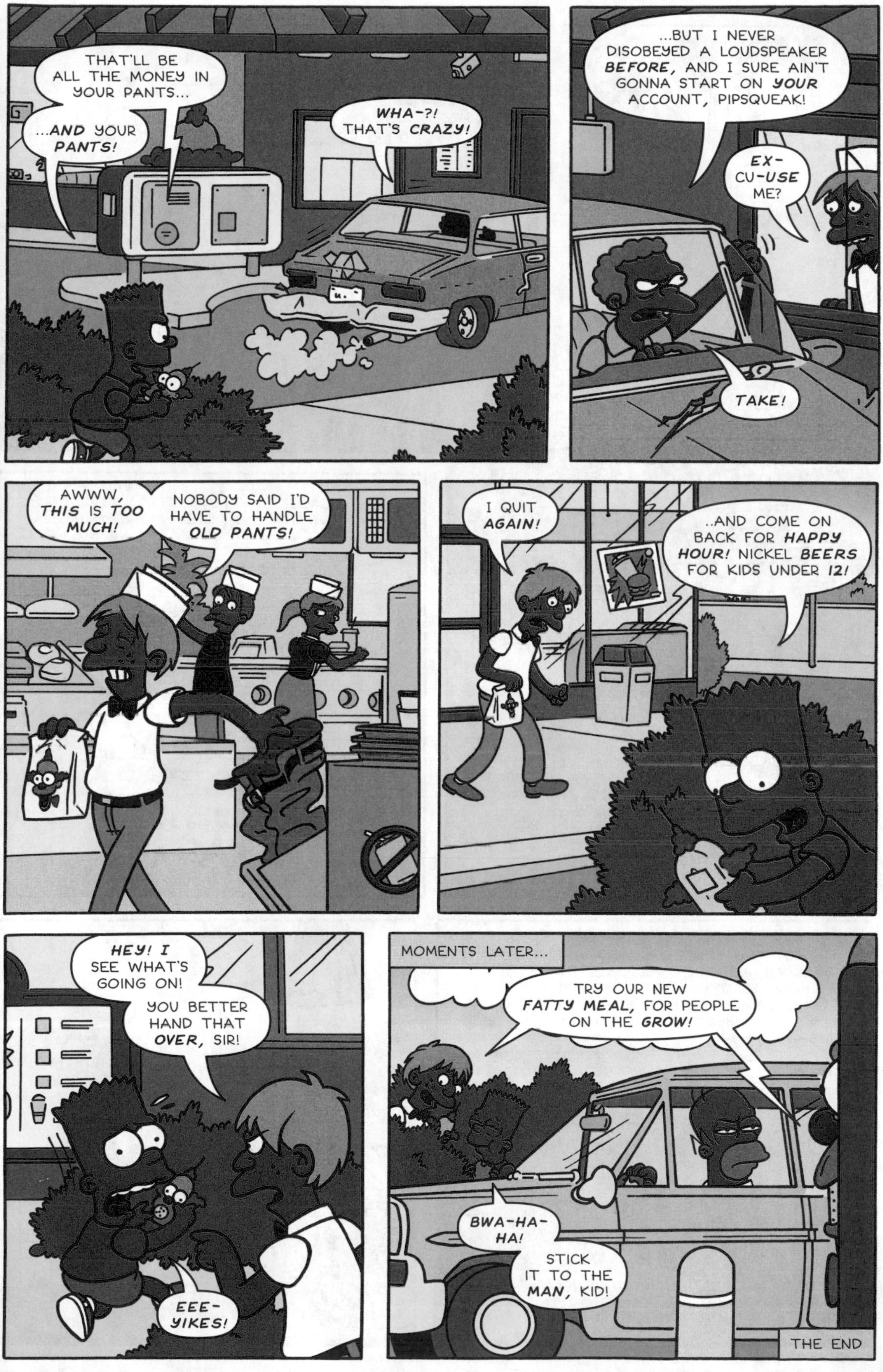
THAT'LL BE ALL THE MONEY IN YOUR PANTS...
...AND YOUR PANTS!
WHA-?! THAT'S CRAZY!
...BUT I NEVER DISOBEYED A LOUDSPEAKER BEFORE, AND I SURE AIN'T GONNA START ON YOUR ACCOUNT, PIPSQUEAK!
EX-CU-USE ME?
TAKE!
AWWW, THIS IS TOO MUCH!
NOBODY SAID I'D HAVE TO HANDLE OLD PANTS!
I QUIT AGAIN!
..AND COME ON BACK FOR HAPPY HOUR! NICKEL BEERS FOR KIDS UNDER 12!
HEY! I SEE WHAT'S GOING ON!
YOU BETTER HAND THAT OVER, SIR!
EEE-YIKES!
MOMENTS LATER...
TRY OUR NEW FATTY MEAL, FOR PEOPLE ON THE GROW!
BWA-HA-HA!
STICK IT TO THE MAN, KID!
THE END

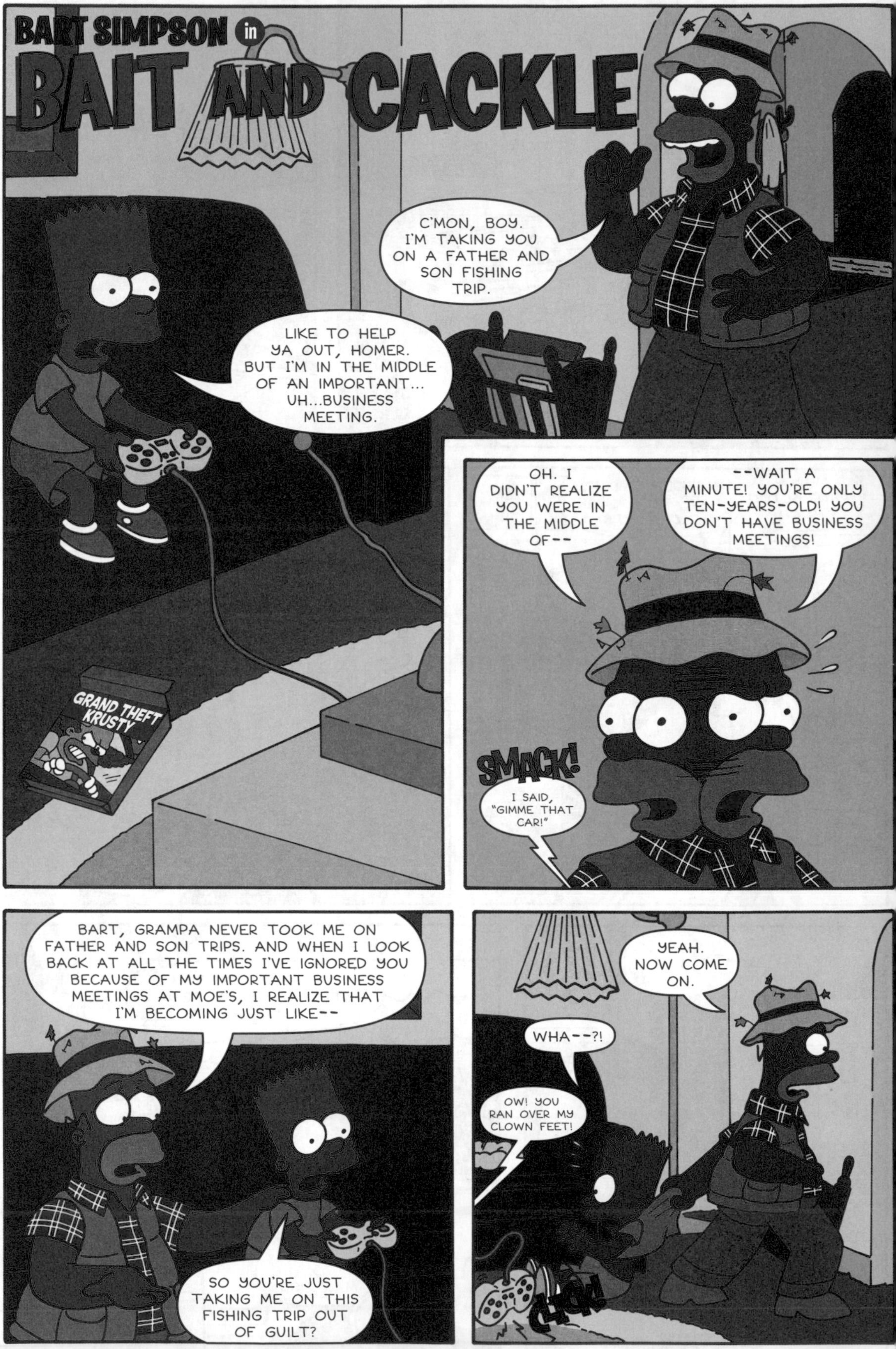
BART SIMPSON in
BAIT AND CACKLE
C'MON, BOY. I'M TAKING YOU ON A FATHER AND SON FISHING TRIP.
LIKE TO HELP YA OUT, HOMER. BUT I'M IN THE MIDDLE OF AN IMPORTANT... UH...BUSINESS MEETING.
GRAND THEFT KRUSTY
OH. I DIDN'T REALIZE YOU WERE IN THE MIDDLE OF--
--WAIT A MINUTE! YOU'RE ONLY TEN-YEARS-OLD! YOU DON'T HAVE BUSINESS MEETINGS!
SMACK!
I SAID, "GIMME THAT CAR!"
BART, GRAMPA NEVER TOOK ME ON FATHER AND SON TRIPS. AND WHEN I LOOK BACK AT ALL THE TIMES I'VE IGNORED YOU BECAUSE OF MY IMPORTANT BUSINESS MEETINGS AT MOE'S, I REALIZE THAT I'M BECOMING JUST LIKE--
SO YOU'RE JUST TAKING ME ON THIS FISHING TRIP OUT OF GUILT?
YEAH. NOW COME ON.
WHA--?!
OW! YOU RAN OVER MY CLOWN FEET!

TONY DIGEROLAMO STORY | *PHIL ORTIZ* PENCILS | *PATRICK OWSLEY* INKS | *NATHAN HAMILL* COLORS | *KAREN BATES* LETTERS | *BILL MORRISON* EDITOR

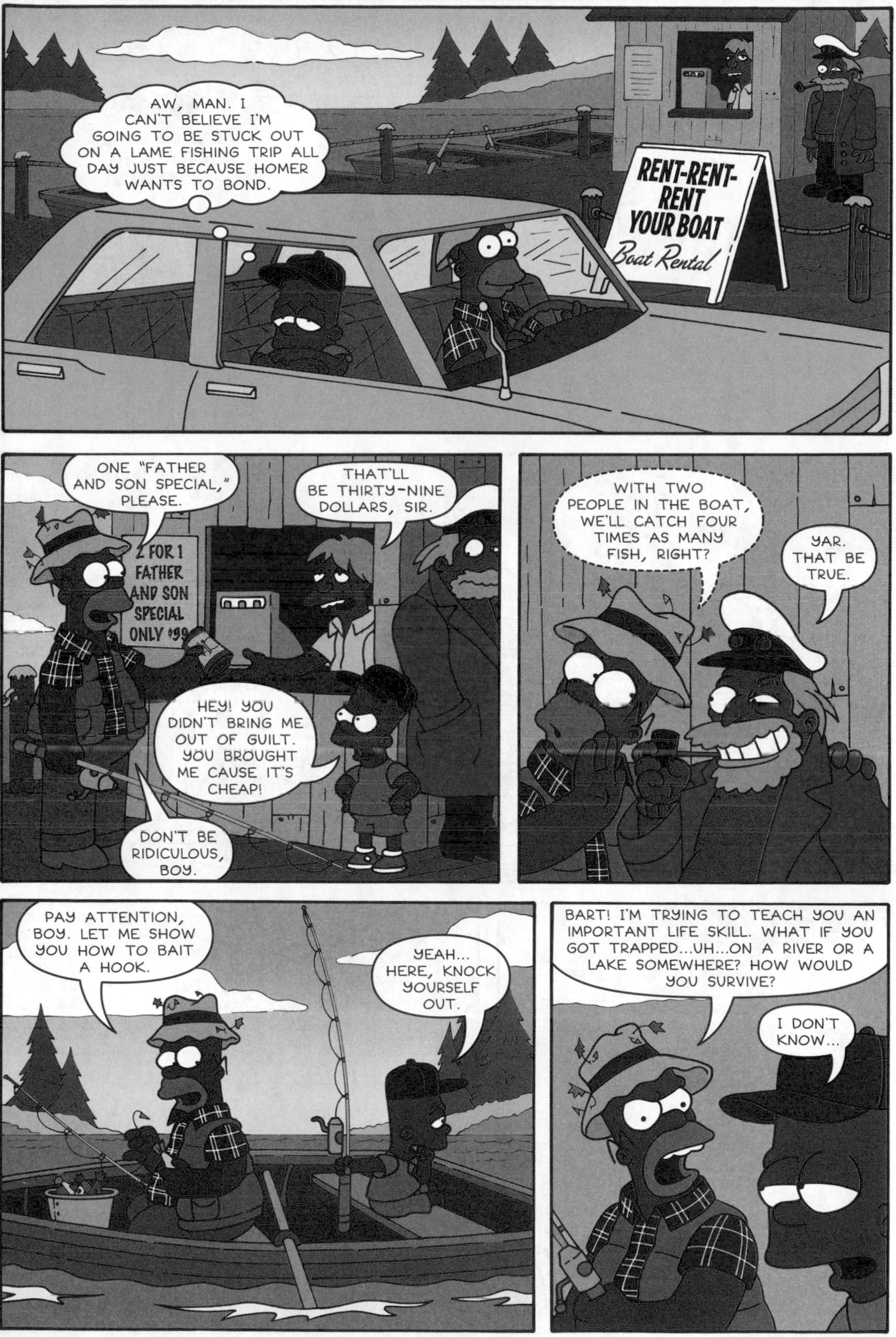
AW, MAN. I CAN'T BELIEVE I'M GOING TO BE STUCK OUT ON A LAME FISHING TRIP ALL DAY JUST BECAUSE HOMER WANTS TO BOND.
RENT-RENT-RENT YOUR BOAT
Boat Rental
ONE "FATHER AND SON SPECIAL," PLEASE.
2 FOR 1 FATHER AND SON SPECIAL ONLY $99
THAT'LL BE THIRTY-NINE DOLLARS, SIR.
HEY! YOU DIDN'T BRING ME OUT OF GUILT. YOU BROUGHT ME CAUSE IT'S CHEAP!
DON'T BE RIDICULOUS, BOY.
WITH TWO PEOPLE IN THE BOAT, WE'LL CATCH FOUR TIMES AS MANY FISH, RIGHT?
YAR. THAT BE TRUE.
PAY ATTENTION, BOY. LET ME SHOW YOU HOW TO BAIT A HOOK.
YEAH... HERE, KNOCK YOURSELF OUT.
BART! I'M TRYING TO TEACH YOU AN IMPORTANT LIFE SKILL. WHAT IF YOU GOT TRAPPED...UH...ON A RIVER OR A LAKE SOMEWHERE? HOW WOULD YOU SURVIVE?
I DON'T KNOW...

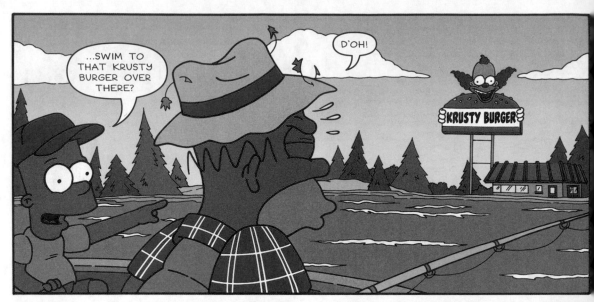

...SWIM TO THAT KRUSTY BURGER OVER THERE?

D'OH!

KRUSTY BURGER

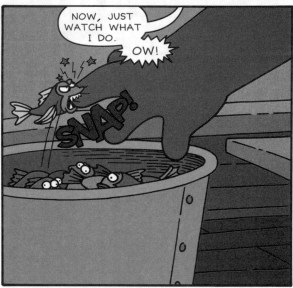

NOW, JUST WATCH WHAT I DO.

OW!

SNAP!

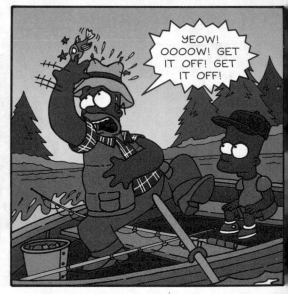

YEOW! OOOOW! GET IT OFF! GET IT OFF!

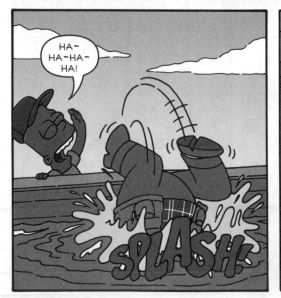

HA-HA-HA-HA!

SPLASH!

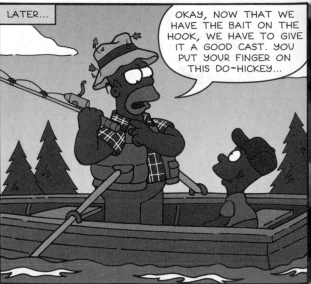

LATER...

OKAY, NOW THAT WE HAVE THE BAIT ON THE HOOK, WE HAVE TO GIVE IT A GOOD CAST. YOU PUT YOUR FINGER ON THIS DO-HICKEY...

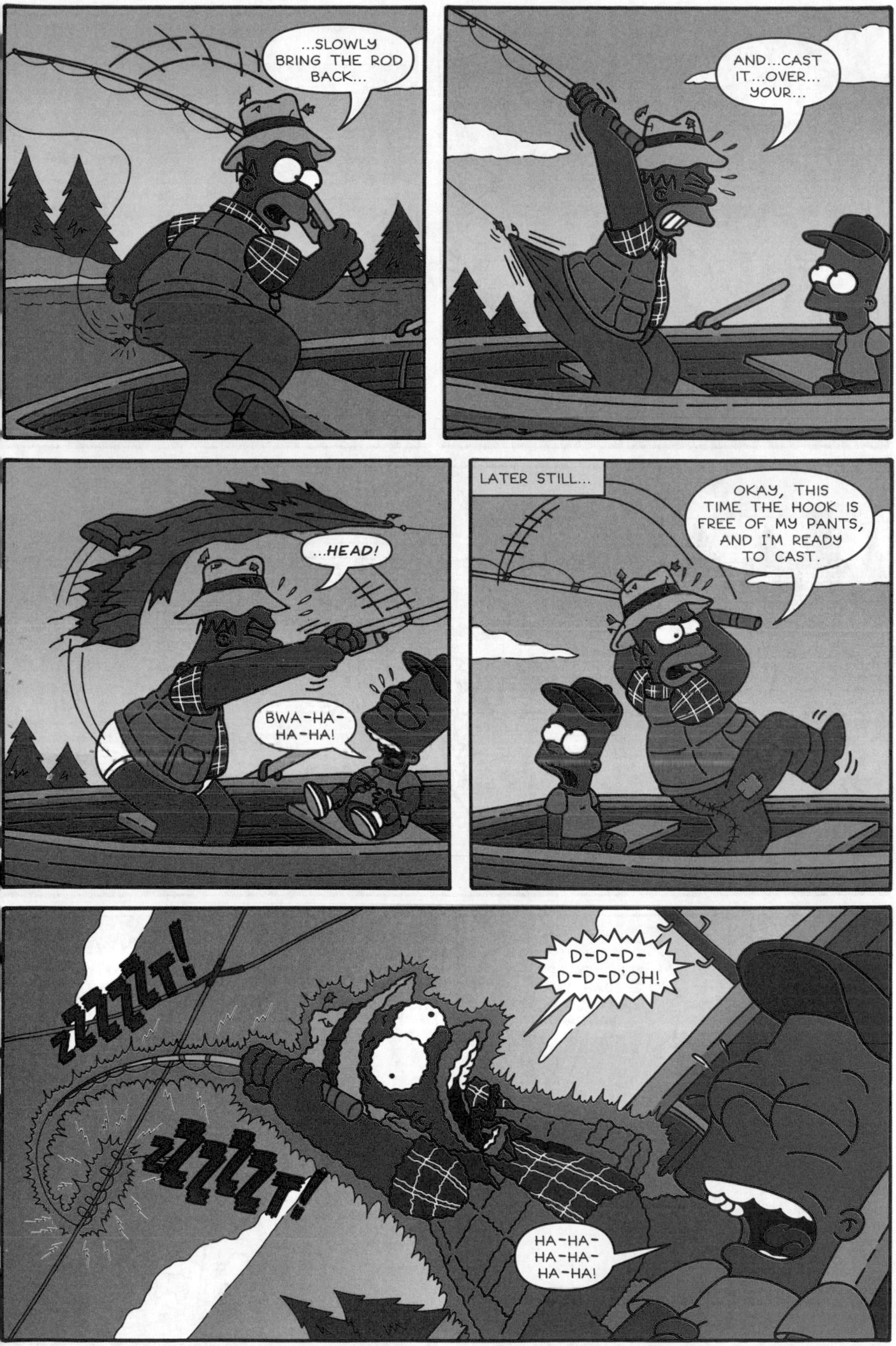
...SLOWLY BRING THE ROD BACK...
AND...CAST IT...OVER... YOUR...
...HEAD!
BWA-HA-HA-HA!
LATER STILL...
OKAY, THIS TIME THE HOOK IS FREE OF MY PANTS, AND I'M READY TO CAST.
ZZZZZT!
ZZZZZZT!
D-D-D-D-D-D'OH!
HA-HA-HA-HA-HA-HA!

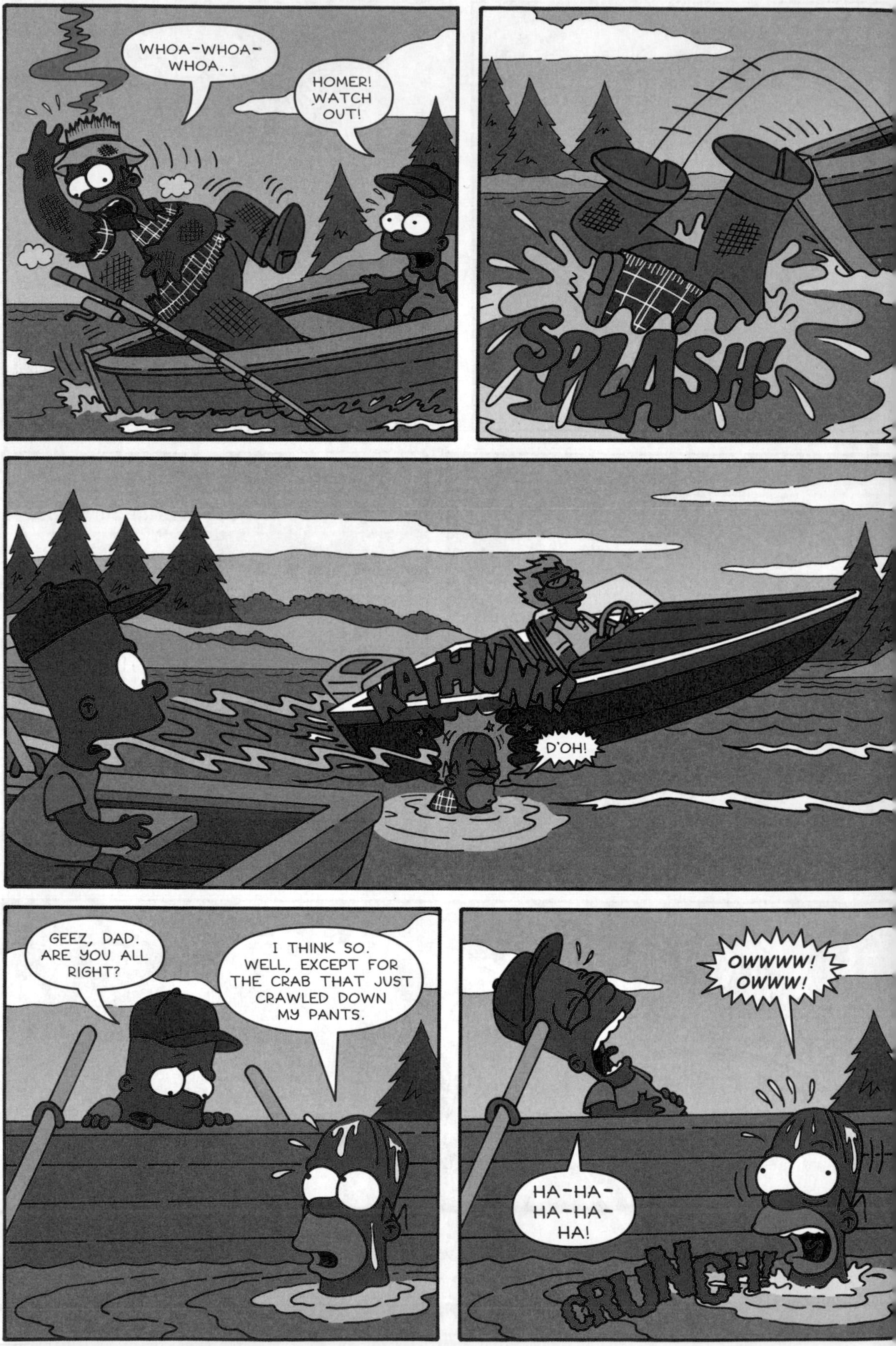
WHOA-WHOA-WHOA...
HOMER! WATCH OUT!
SPLASH!
KATHUNK!
D'OH!
GEEZ, DAD. ARE YOU ALL RIGHT?
I THINK SO. WELL, EXCEPT FOR THE CRAB THAT JUST CRAWLED DOWN MY PANTS.
OWWWW! OWWW!
HA-HA-HA-HA-HA!
CRUNCH!

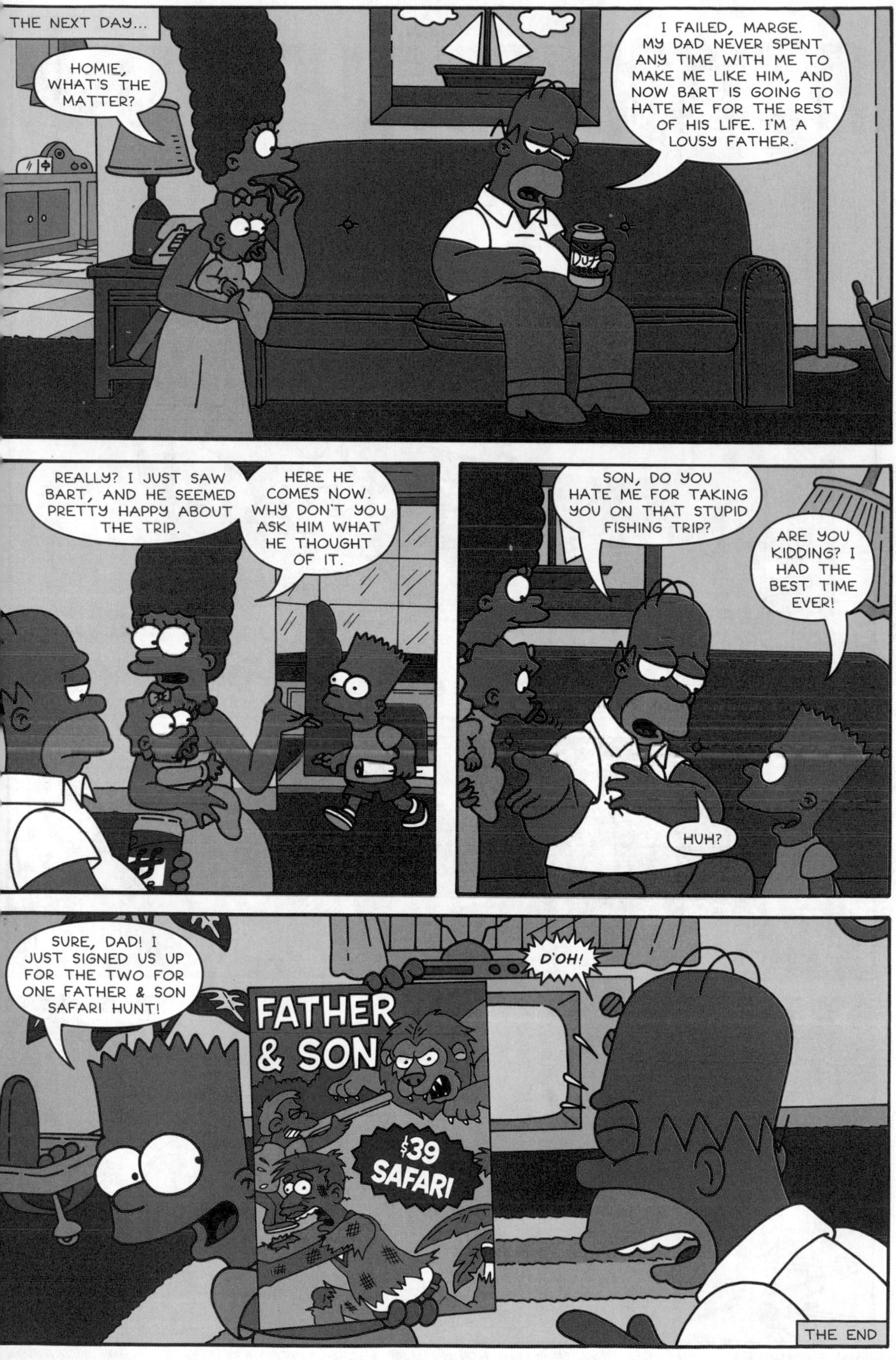
THE NEXT DAY...
HOMIE, WHAT'S THE MATTER?
I FAILED, MARGE. MY DAD NEVER SPENT ANY TIME WITH ME TO MAKE ME LIKE HIM, AND NOW BART IS GOING TO HATE ME FOR THE REST OF HIS LIFE. I'M A LOUSY FATHER.
REALLY? I JUST SAW BART, AND HE SEEMED PRETTY HAPPY ABOUT THE TRIP.
HERE HE COMES NOW. WHY DON'T YOU ASK HIM WHAT HE THOUGHT OF IT.
SON, DO YOU HATE ME FOR TAKING YOU ON THAT STUPID FISHING TRIP?
ARE YOU KIDDING? I HAD THE BEST TIME EVER!
HUH?
SURE, DAD! I JUST SIGNED US UP FOR THE TWO FOR ONE FATHER & SON SAFARI HUNT!
D'OH!
FATHER & SON
$39 SAFARI
THE END

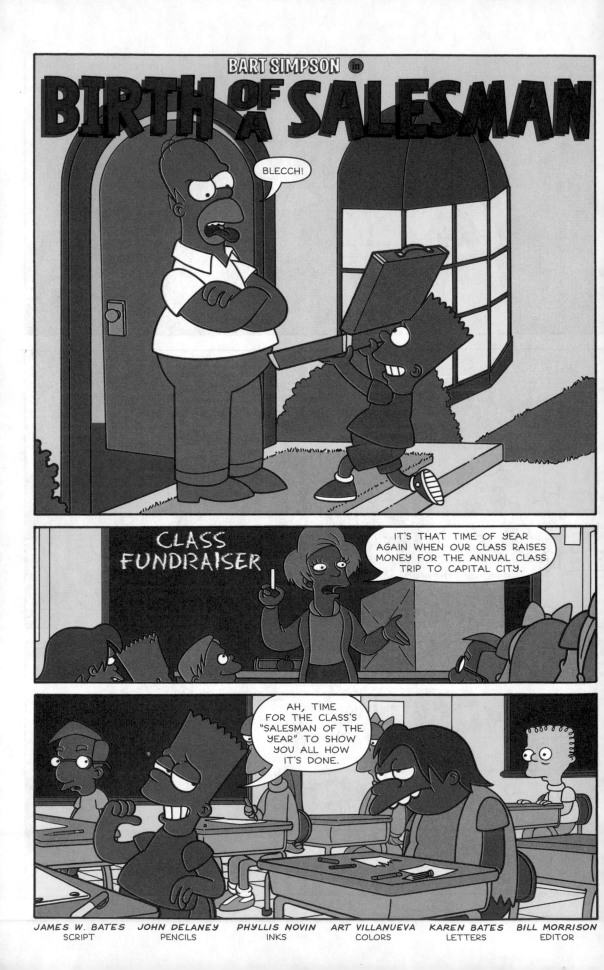

BART SIMPSON in

BIRTH OF A SALESMAN

BLECCH!

CLASS FUNDRAISER

IT'S THAT TIME OF YEAR AGAIN WHEN OUR CLASS RAISES MONEY FOR THE ANNUAL CLASS TRIP TO CAPITAL CITY.

AH, TIME FOR THE CLASS'S "SALESMAN OF THE YEAR" TO SHOW YOU ALL HOW IT'S DONE.

JAMES W. BATES
SCRIPT

JOHN DELANEY
PENCILS

PHYLLIS NOVIN
INKS

ART VILLANUEVA
COLORS

KAREN BATES
LETTERS

BILL MORRISON
EDITOR

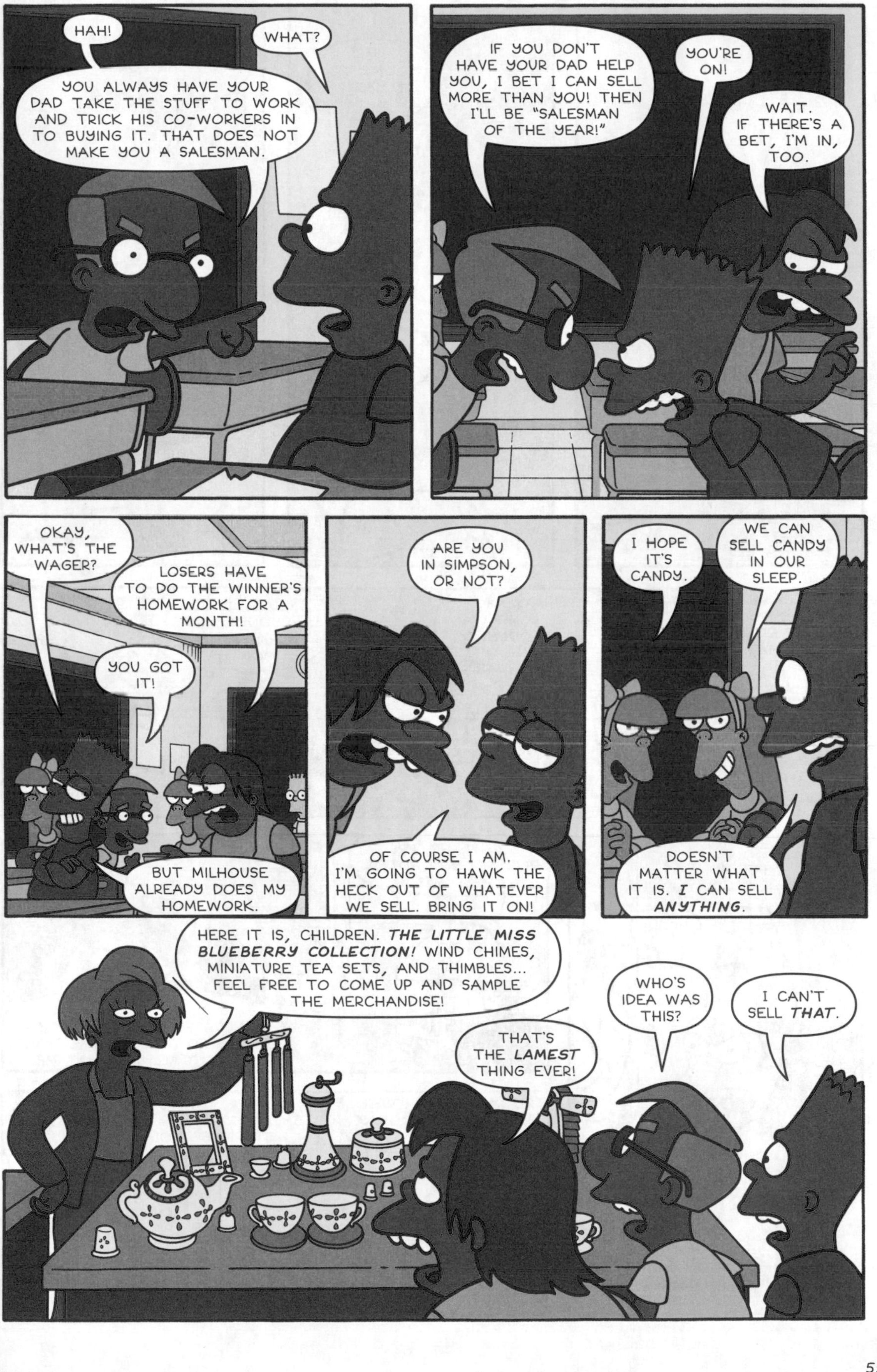
HAH!
YOU ALWAYS HAVE YOUR DAD TAKE THE STUFF TO WORK AND TRICK HIS CO-WORKERS IN TO BUYING IT. THAT DOES NOT MAKE YOU A SALESMAN.
WHAT?
IF YOU DON'T HAVE YOUR DAD HELP YOU, I BET I CAN SELL MORE THAN YOU! THEN I'LL BE "SALESMAN OF THE YEAR!"
YOU'RE ON!
WAIT. IF THERE'S A BET, I'M IN, TOO.
OKAY, WHAT'S THE WAGER?
LOSERS HAVE TO DO THE WINNER'S HOMEWORK FOR A MONTH!
YOU GOT IT!
BUT MILHOUSE ALREADY DOES MY HOMEWORK.
ARE YOU IN SIMPSON, OR NOT?
OF COURSE I AM. I'M GOING TO HAWK THE HECK OUT OF WHATEVER WE SELL. BRING IT ON!
I HOPE IT'S CANDY.
WE CAN SELL CANDY IN OUR SLEEP.
DOESN'T MATTER WHAT IT IS. *I* CAN SELL ***ANYTHING***.
HERE IT IS, CHILDREN. ***THE LITTLE MISS BLUEBERRY COLLECTION!*** WIND CHIMES, MINIATURE TEA SETS, AND THIMBLES... FEEL FREE TO COME UP AND SAMPLE THE MERCHANDISE!
THAT'S THE ***LAMEST*** THING EVER!
WHO'S IDEA WAS THIS?
I CAN'T SELL ***THAT***.

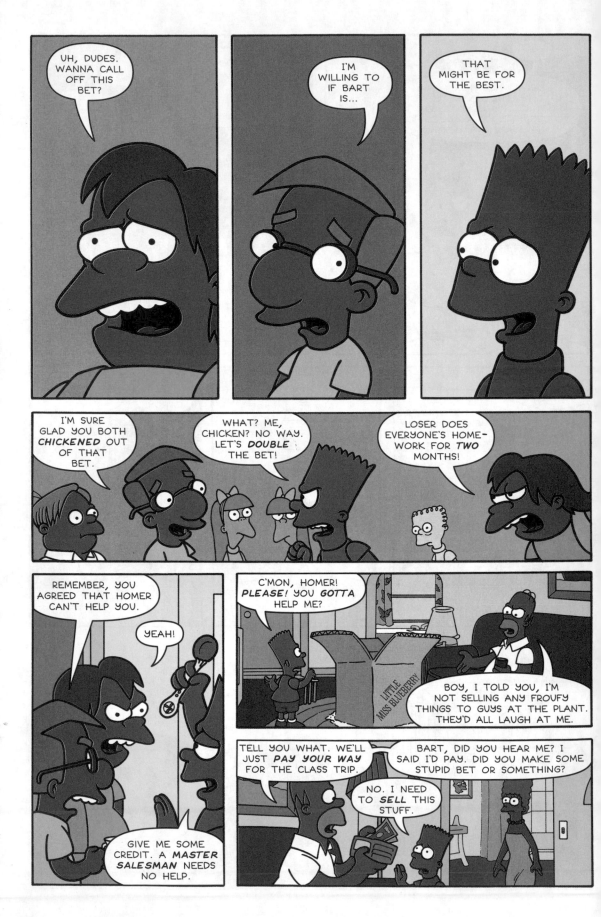

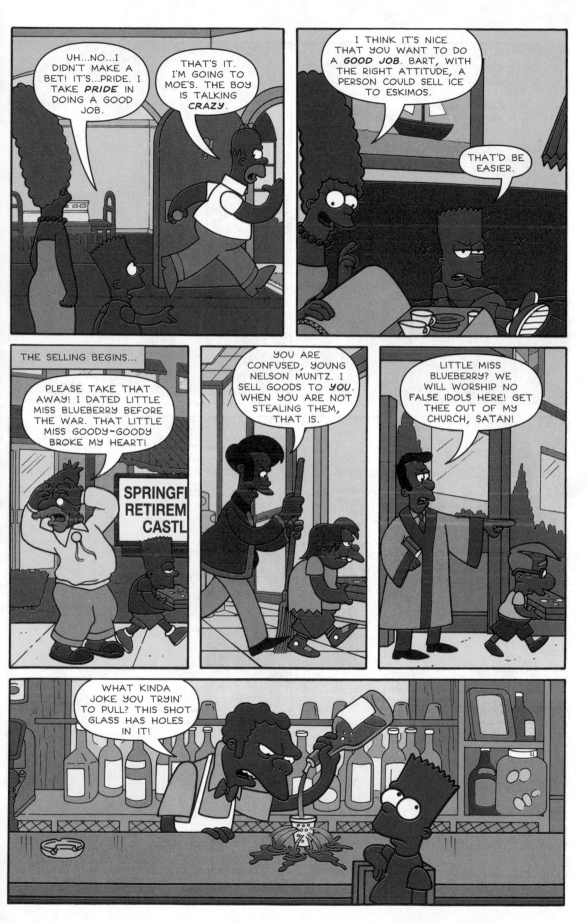

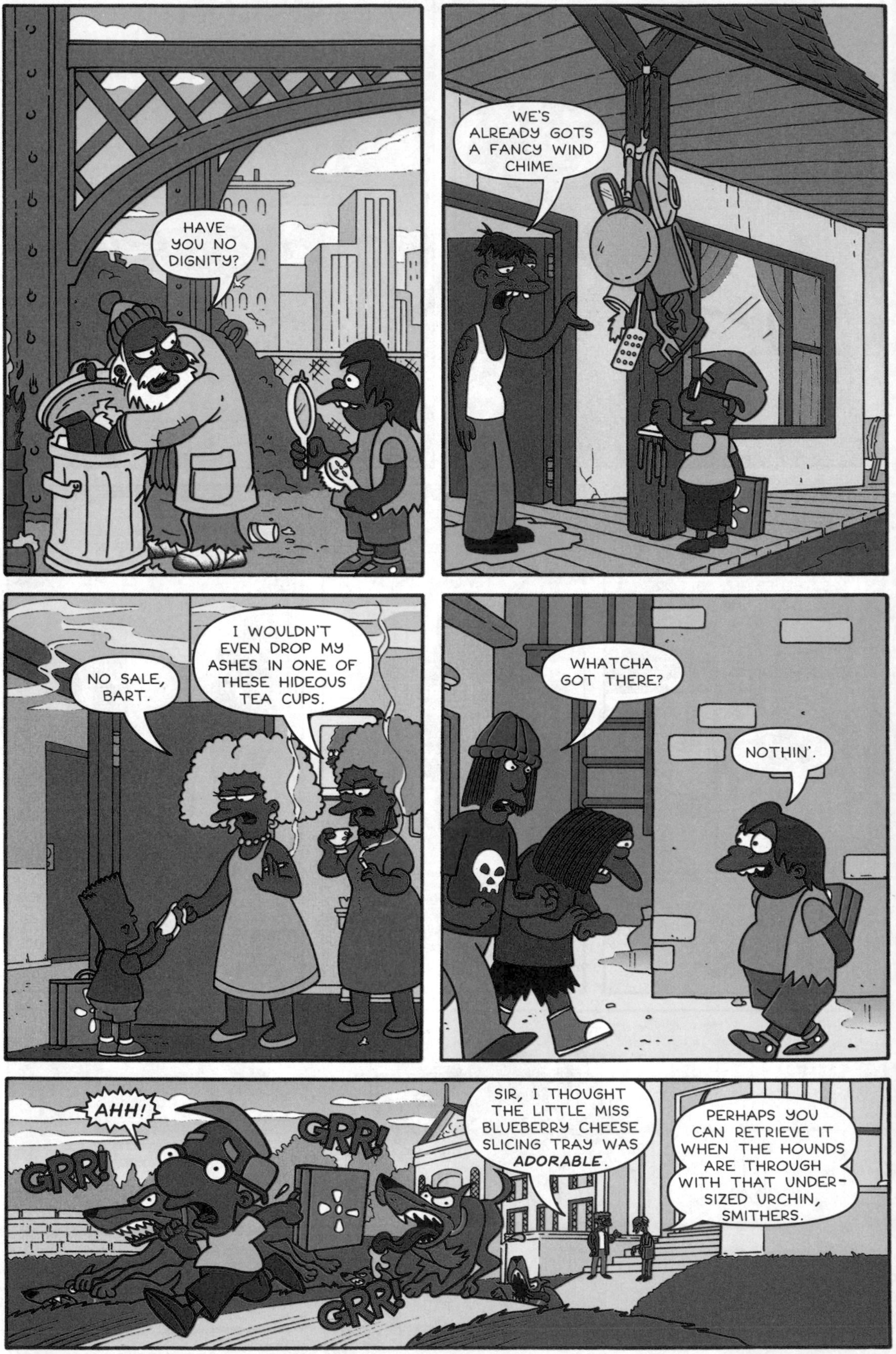
HAVE YOU NO DIGNITY?
WE'S ALREADY GOTS A FANCY WIND CHIME.
NO SALE, BART.
I WOULDN'T EVEN DROP MY ASHES IN ONE OF THESE HIDEOUS TEA CUPS.
WHATCHA GOT THERE?
NOTHIN'.
AHH!
GRR!
GRR!
GRR!
SIR, I THOUGHT THE LITTLE MISS BLUEBERRY CHEESE SLICING TRAY WAS ADORABLE.
PERHAPS YOU CAN RETRIEVE IT WHEN THE HOUNDS ARE THROUGH WITH THAT UNDER-SIZED URCHIN, SMITHERS.

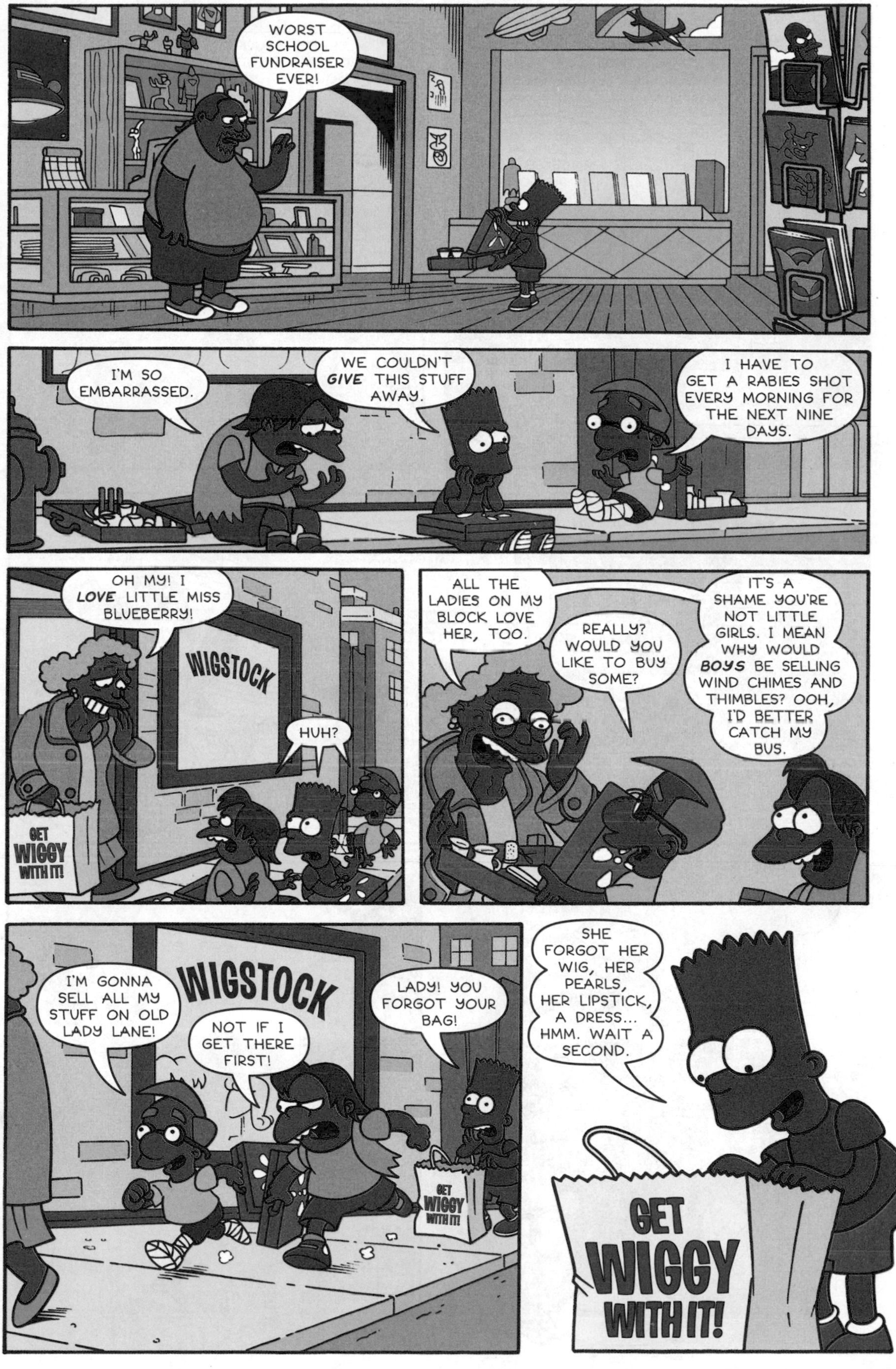
WORST SCHOOL FUNDRAISER EVER!
I'M SO EMBARRASSED.
WE COULDN'T GIVE THIS STUFF AWAY.
I HAVE TO GET A RABIES SHOT EVERY MORNING FOR THE NEXT NINE DAYS.
OH MY! I LOVE LITTLE MISS BLUEBERRY!
WIGSTOCK
HUH?
GET WIGGY WITH IT!
ALL THE LADIES ON MY BLOCK LOVE HER, TOO.
REALLY? WOULD YOU LIKE TO BUY SOME?
IT'S A SHAME YOU'RE NOT LITTLE GIRLS. I MEAN WHY WOULD BOYS BE SELLING WIND CHIMES AND THIMBLES? OOH, I'D BETTER CATCH MY BUS.
WIGSTOCK
I'M GONNA SELL ALL MY STUFF ON OLD LADY LANE!
NOT IF I GET THERE FIRST!
LADY! YOU FORGOT YOUR BAG!
GET WIGGY WITH IT!
SHE FORGOT HER WIG, HER PEARLS, HER LIPSTICK, A DRESS... HMM. WAIT A SECOND.
GET WIGGY WITH IT!

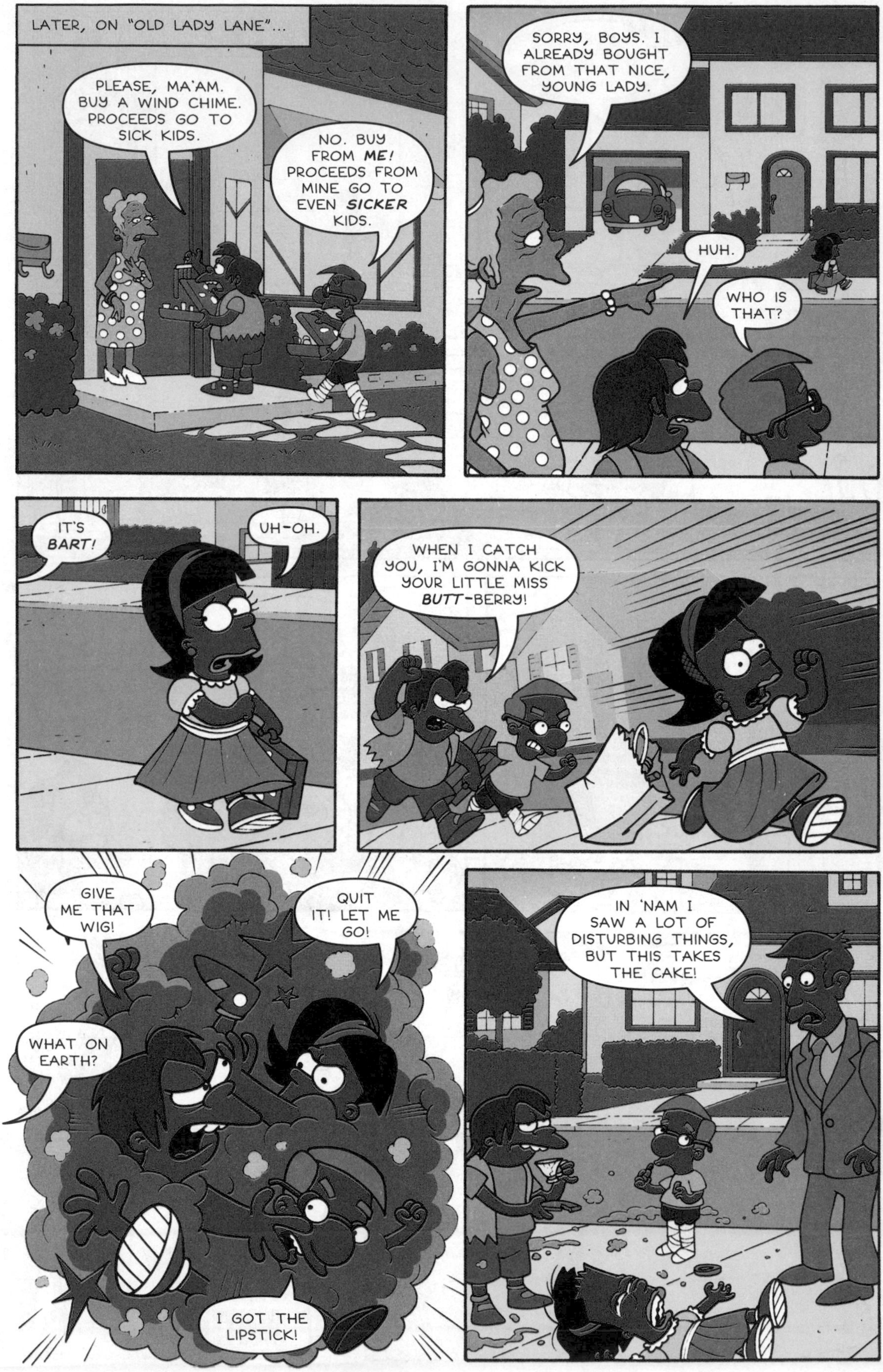
LATER, ON "OLD LADY LANE"...
PLEASE, MA'AM. BUY A WIND CHIME. PROCEEDS GO TO SICK KIDS.
NO. BUY FROM ME! PROCEEDS FROM MINE GO TO EVEN SICKER KIDS.
SORRY, BOYS. I ALREADY BOUGHT FROM THAT NICE, YOUNG LADY.
HUH.
WHO IS THAT?
IT'S BART!
UH-OH.
WHEN I CATCH YOU, I'M GONNA KICK YOUR LITTLE MISS BUTT-BERRY!
GIVE ME THAT WIG!
QUIT IT! LET ME GO!
WHAT ON EARTH?
I GOT THE LIPSTICK!
IN 'NAM I SAW A LOT OF DISTURBING THINGS, BUT THIS TAKES THE CAKE!

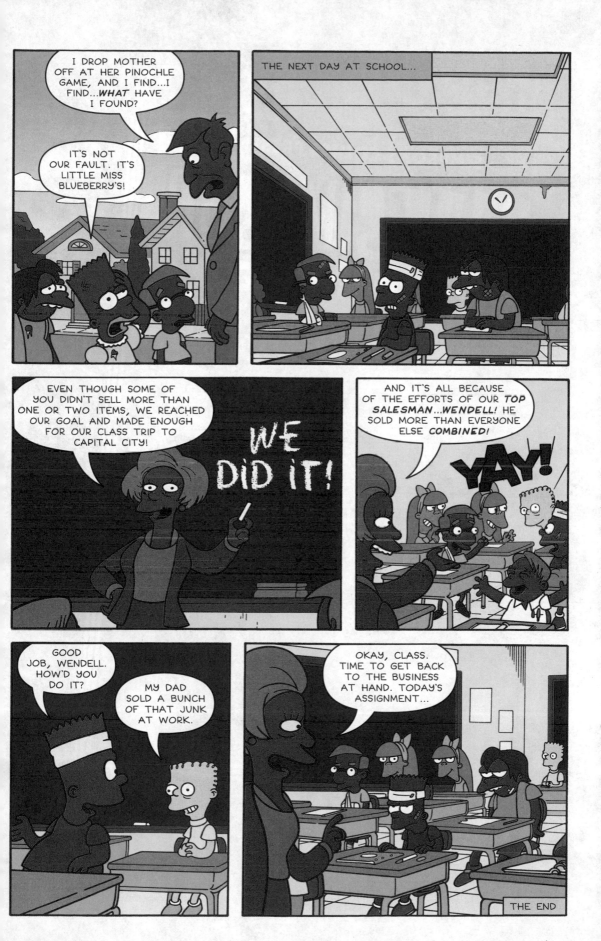

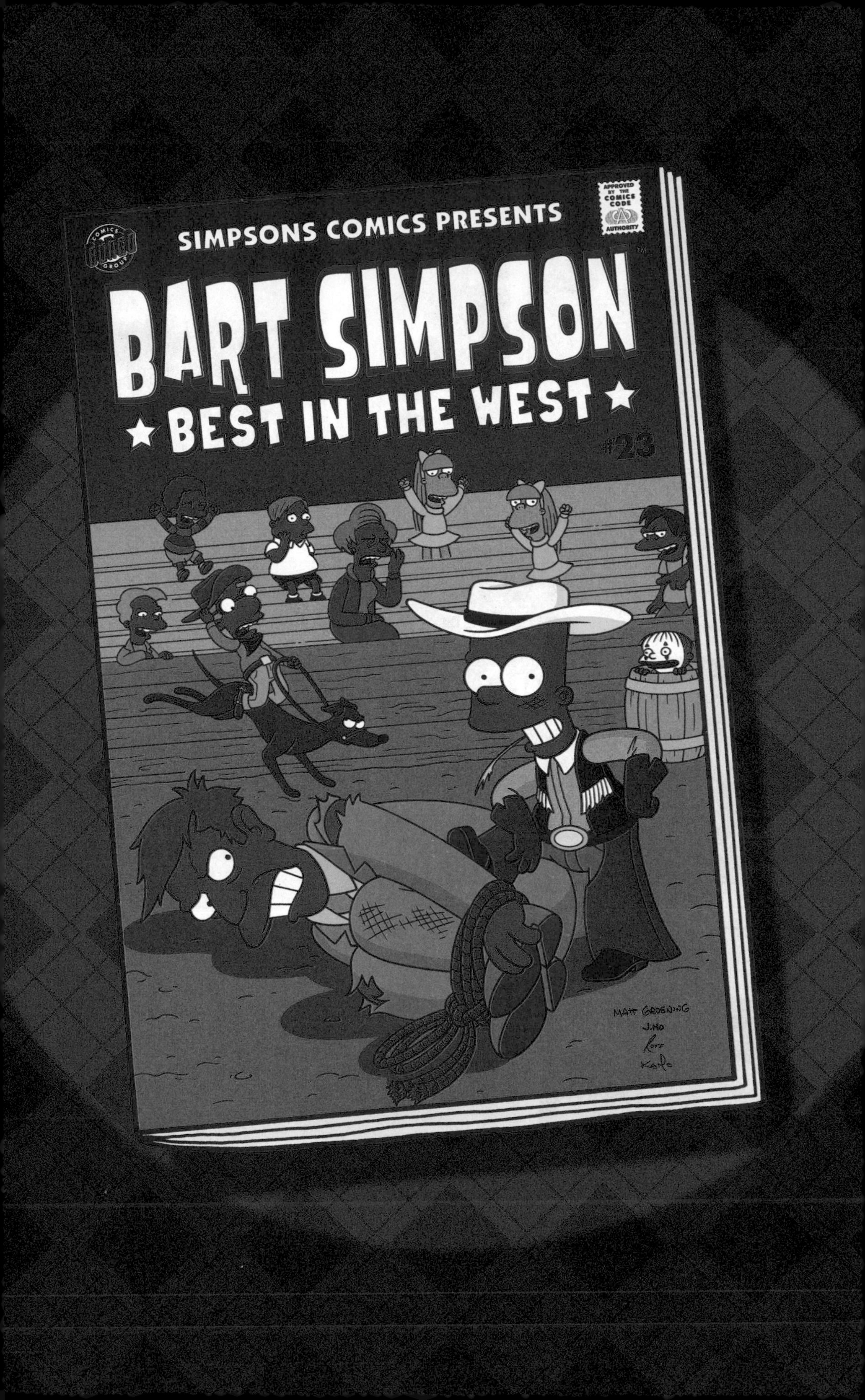

SIMPSONS COMICS PRESENTS
BART SIMPSON
★ BEST IN THE WEST ★
#23
APPROVED BY THE COMICS CODE AUTHORITY

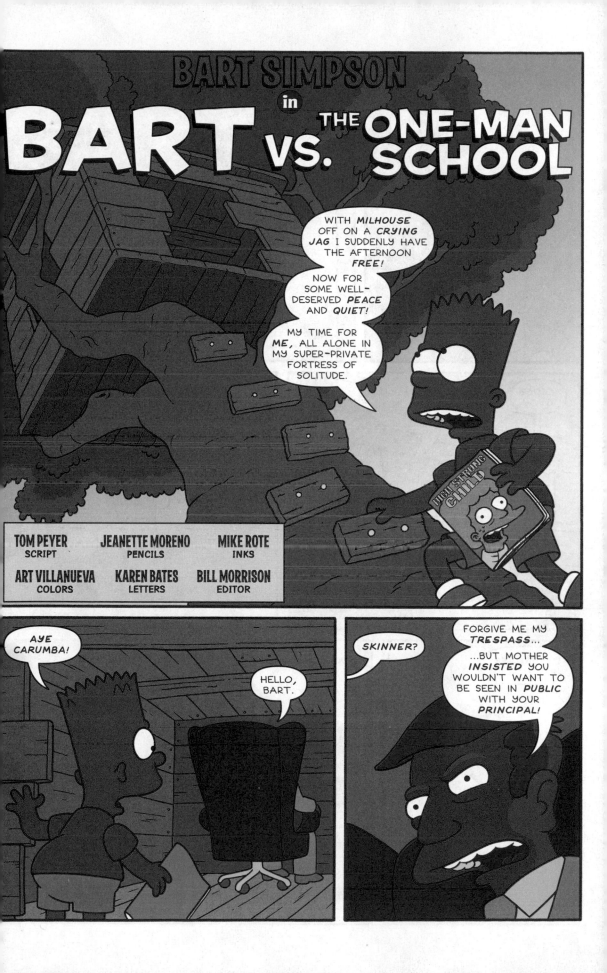

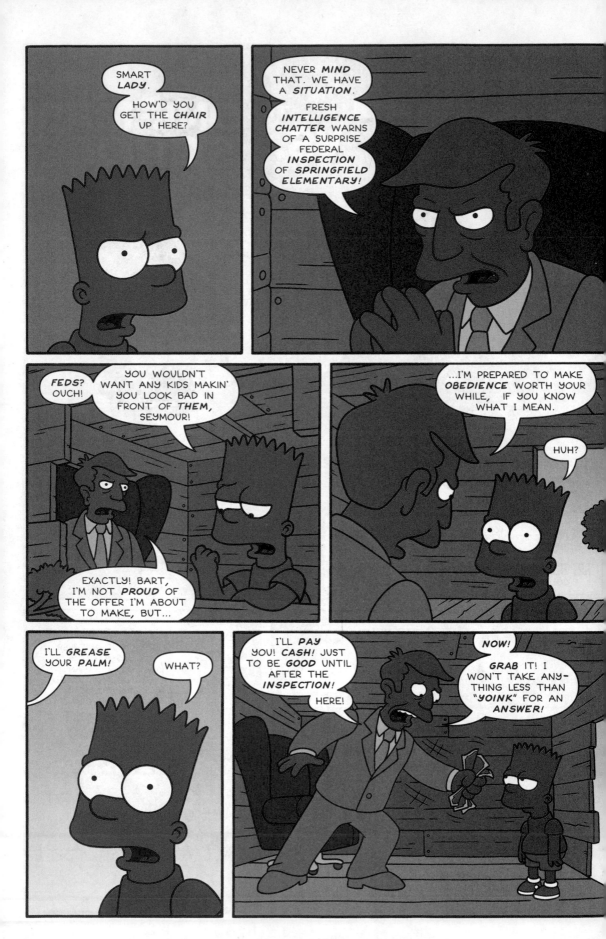

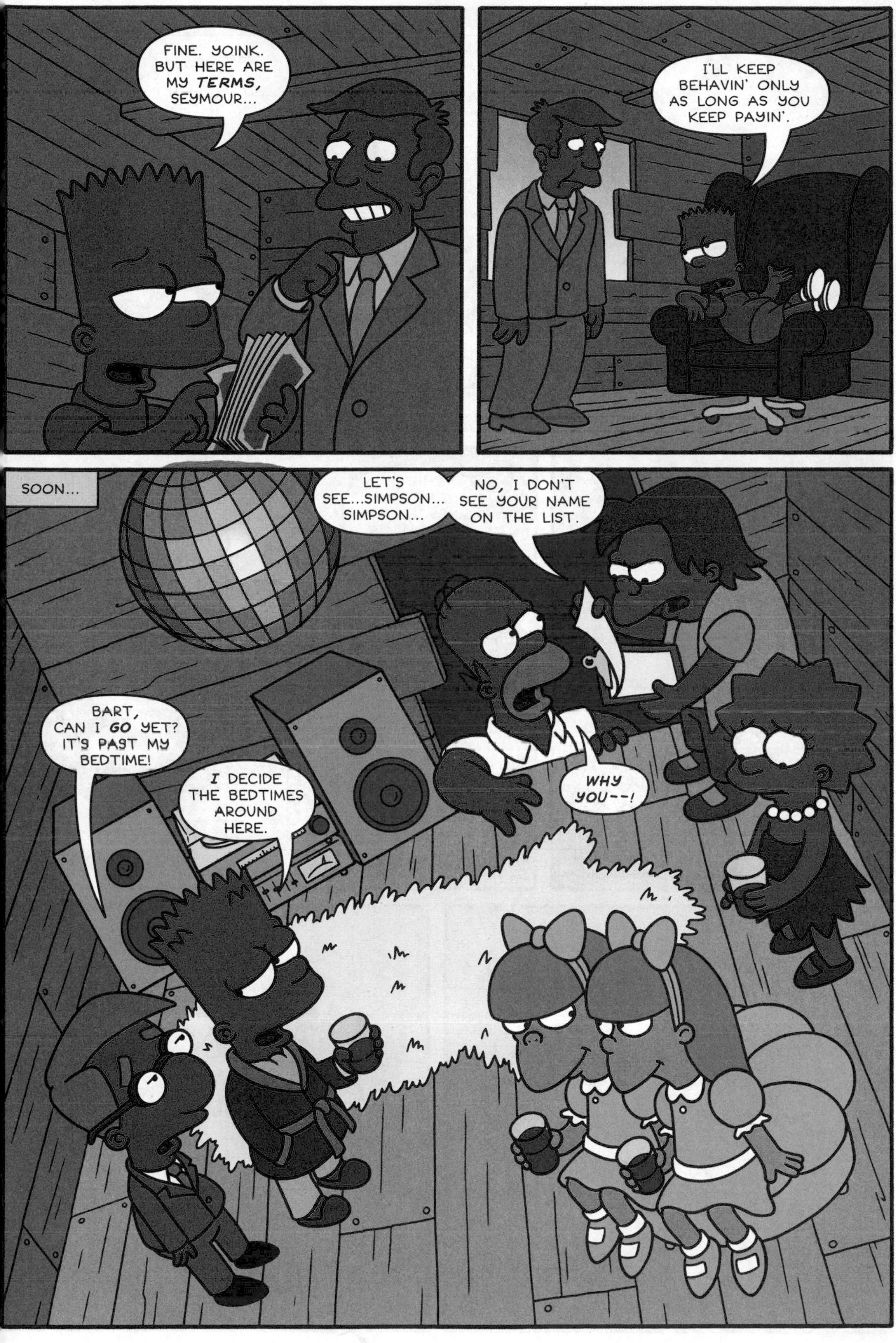
FINE. YOINK. BUT HERE ARE MY *TERMS,* SEYMOUR...
I'LL KEEP BEHAVIN' ONLY AS LONG AS YOU KEEP PAYIN'.
SOON...
LET'S SEE...SIMPSON... SIMPSON...
NO, I DON'T SEE YOUR NAME ON THE LIST.
WHY YOU--!
BART, CAN I *GO* YET? IT'S PAST MY BEDTIME!
I DECIDE THE BEDTIMES AROUND HERE.

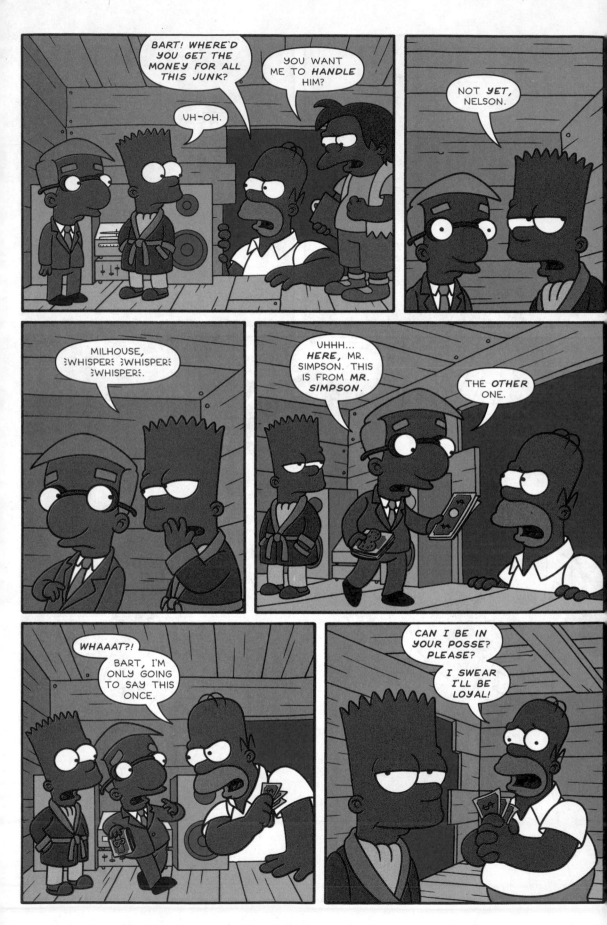

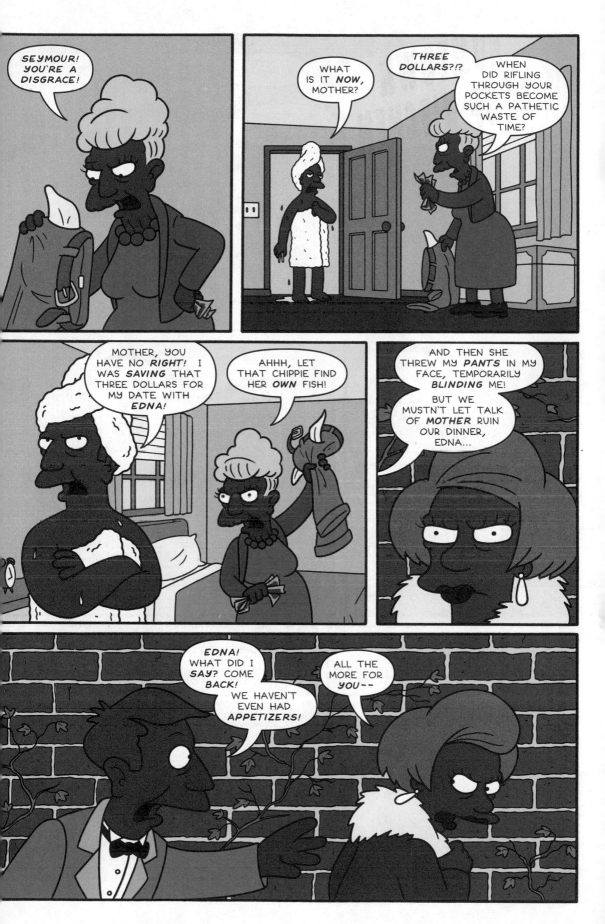

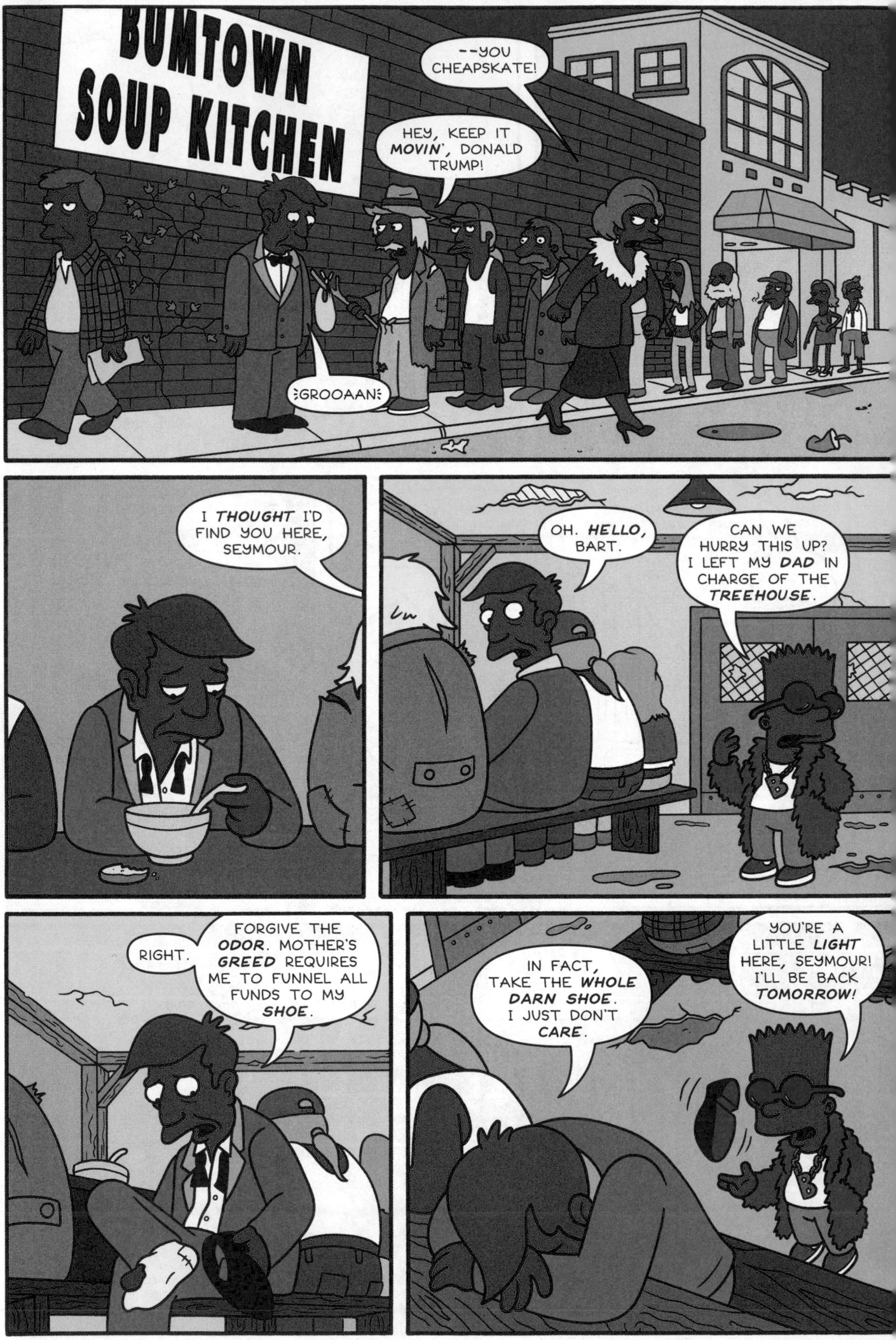
BUMTOWN SOUP KITCHEN
--YOU CHEAPSKATE!
HEY, KEEP IT MOVIN', DONALD TRUMP!
GROOAAN
I THOUGHT I'D FIND YOU HERE, SEYMOUR.
OH. HELLO, BART.
CAN WE HURRY THIS UP? I LEFT MY DAD IN CHARGE OF THE TREEHOUSE.
RIGHT.
FORGIVE THE ODOR. MOTHER'S GREED REQUIRES ME TO FUNNEL ALL FUNDS TO MY SHOE.
IN FACT, TAKE THE WHOLE DARN SHOE. I JUST DON'T CARE.
YOU'RE A LITTLE LIGHT HERE, SEYMOUR! I'LL BE BACK TOMORROW!

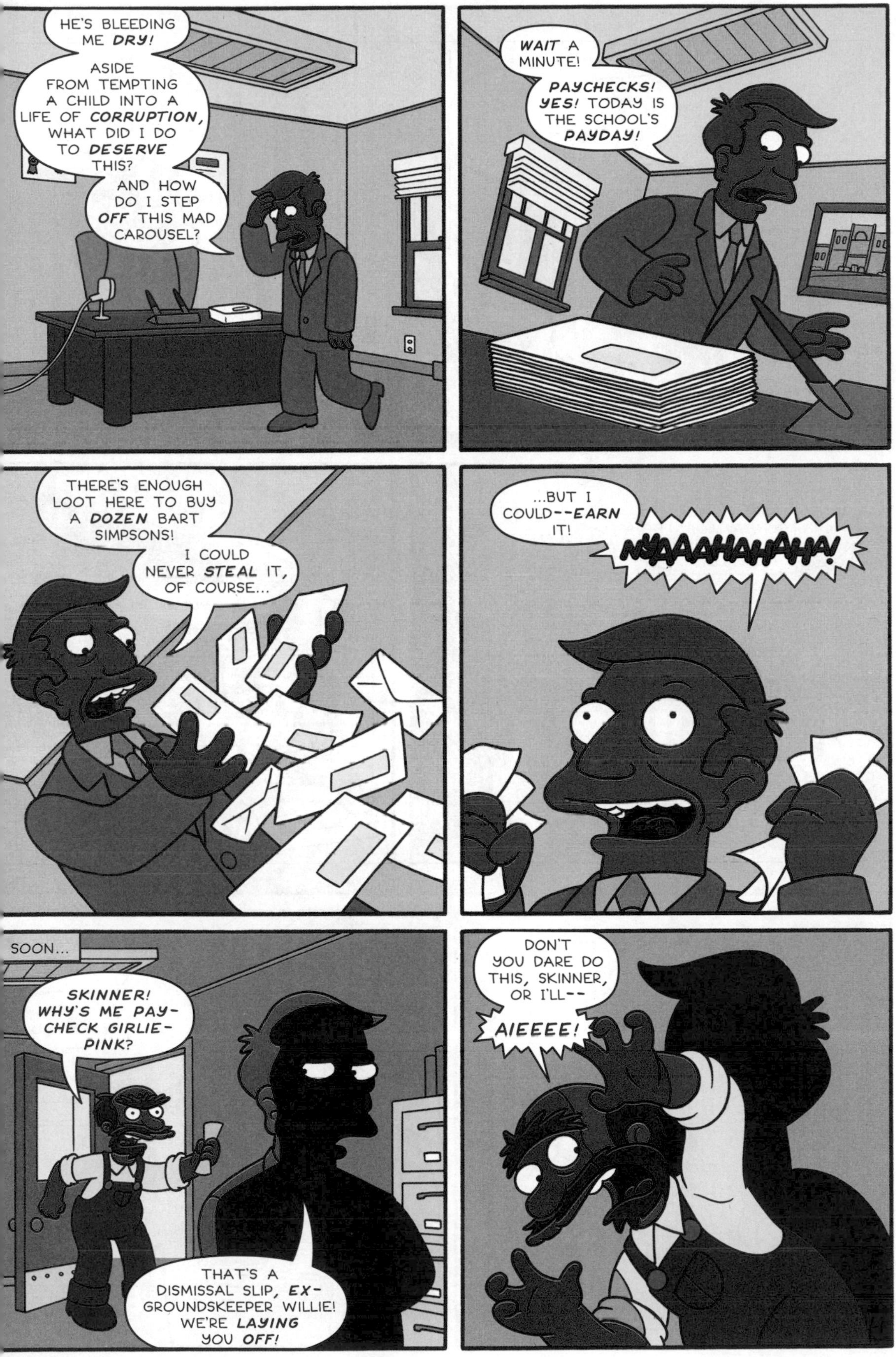
HE'S BLEEDING ME DRY!
ASIDE FROM TEMPTING A CHILD INTO A LIFE OF CORRUPTION, WHAT DID I DO TO DESERVE THIS?
AND HOW DO I STEP OFF THIS MAD CAROUSEL?
WAIT A MINUTE!
PAYCHECKS! YES! TODAY IS THE SCHOOL'S PAYDAY!
THERE'S ENOUGH LOOT HERE TO BUY A DOZEN BART SIMPSONS!
I COULD NEVER STEAL IT, OF COURSE...
...BUT I COULD--EARN IT!
NYAAAHAHAHA!
SOON...
SKINNER! WHY'S ME PAY-CHECK GIRLIE-PINK?
THAT'S A DISMISSAL SLIP, EX-GROUNDSKEEPER WILLIE! WE'RE LAYING YOU OFF!
DON'T YOU DARE DO THIS, SKINNER, OR I'LL--
AIEEEE!

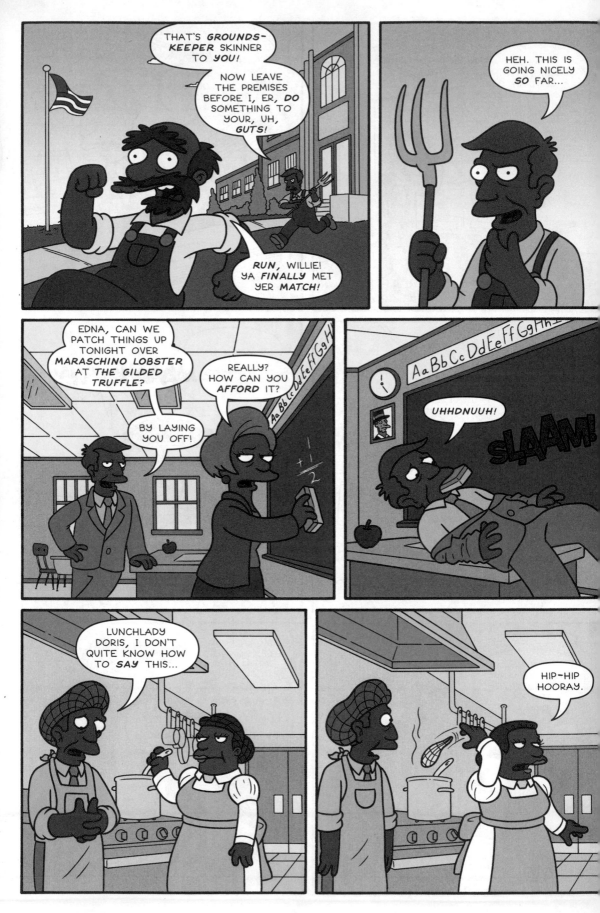

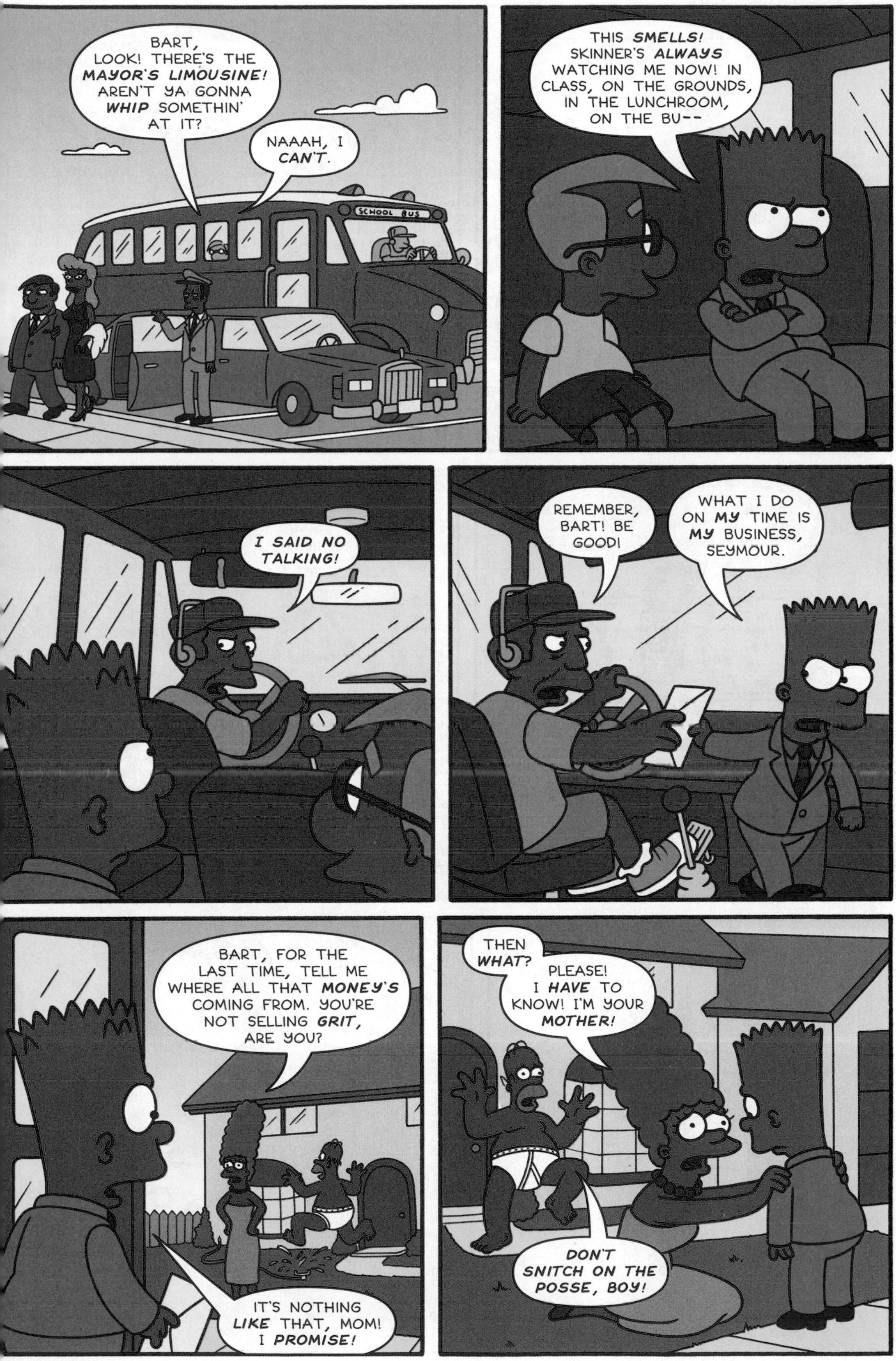
BART, LOOK! THERE'S THE MAYOR'S LIMOUSINE! AREN'T YA GONNA WHIP SOMETHIN' AT IT?
NAAAH, I CAN'T.
SCHOOL BUS
THIS SMELLS! SKINNER'S ALWAYS WATCHING ME NOW! IN CLASS, ON THE GROUNDS, IN THE LUNCHROOM, ON THE BU--
I SAID NO TALKING!
REMEMBER, BART! BE GOOD!
WHAT I DO ON MY TIME IS MY BUSINESS, SEYMOUR.
BART, FOR THE LAST TIME, TELL ME WHERE ALL THAT MONEY'S COMING FROM. YOU'RE NOT SELLING GRIT, ARE YOU?
IT'S NOTHING LIKE THAT, MOM! I PROMISE!
THEN WHAT?
PLEASE! I HAVE TO KNOW! I'M YOUR MOTHER!
DON'T SNITCH ON THE POSSE, BOY!

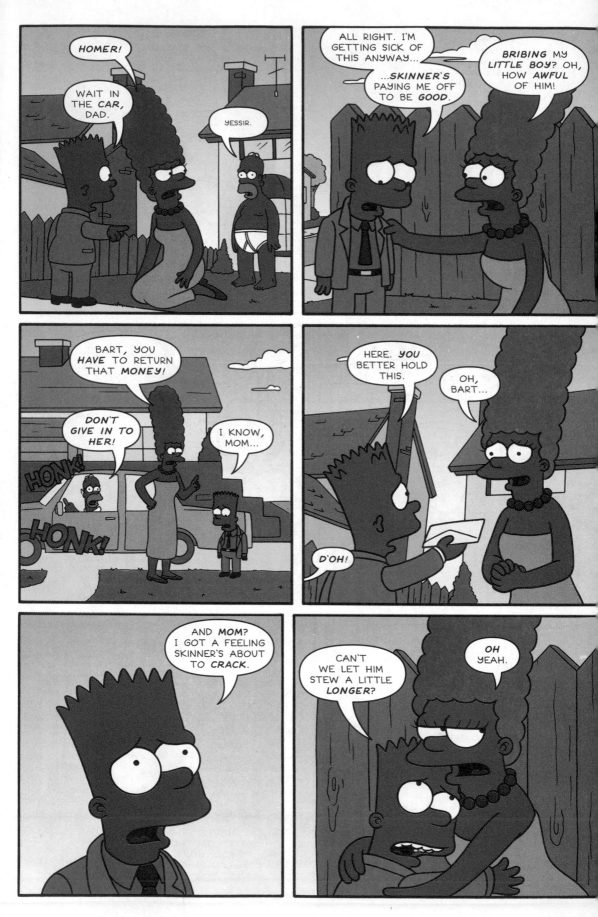

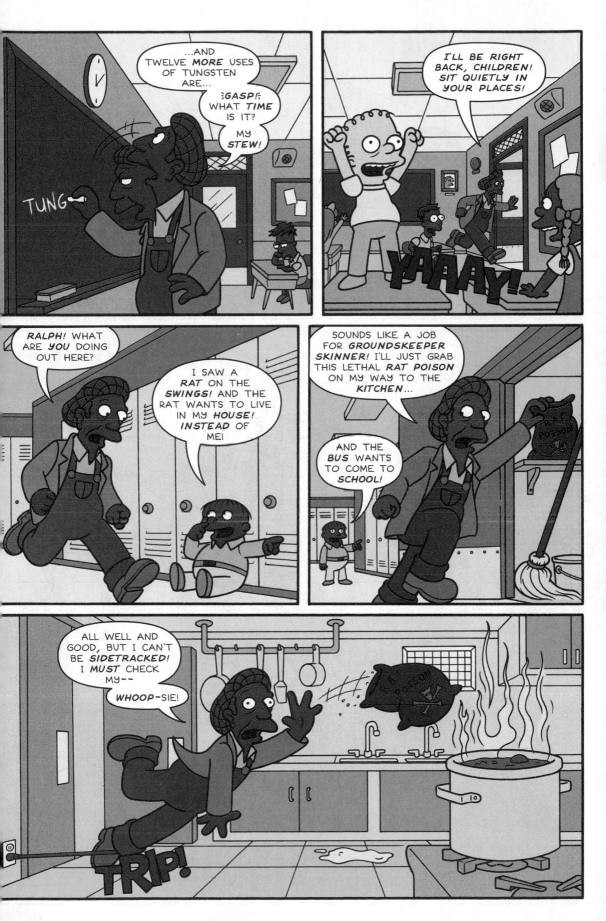

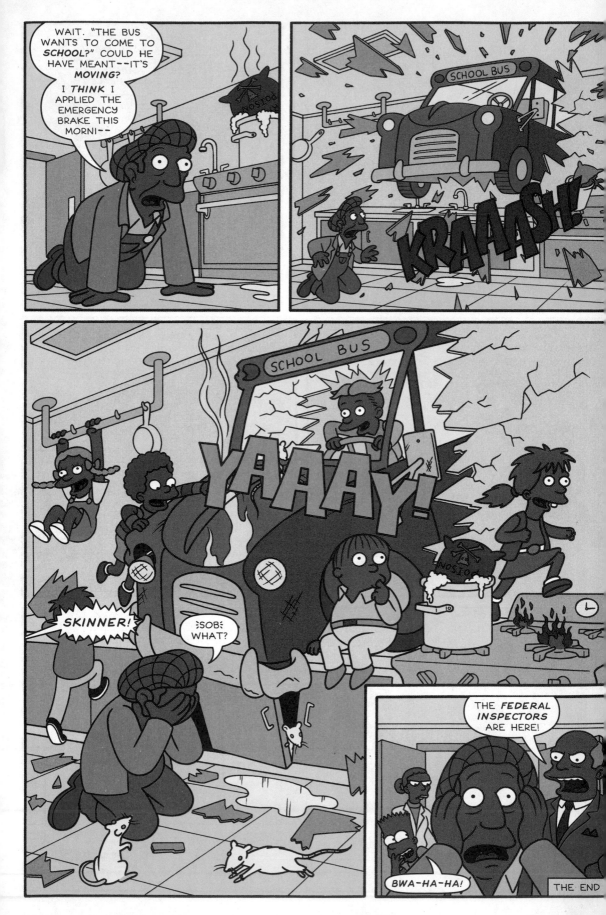

WAIT. "THE BUS WANTS TO COME TO *SCHOOL?*" COULD HE HAVE MEANT--IT'S *MOVING?*

I *THINK* I APPLIED THE EMERGENCY BRAKE THIS MORNI--

SCHOOL BUS

KRAAASH!

SCHOOL BUS

YAAAY!

SKINNER!

:SOB: WHAT?

THE *FEDERAL INSPECTORS* ARE HERE!

BWA-HA-HA!

THE END

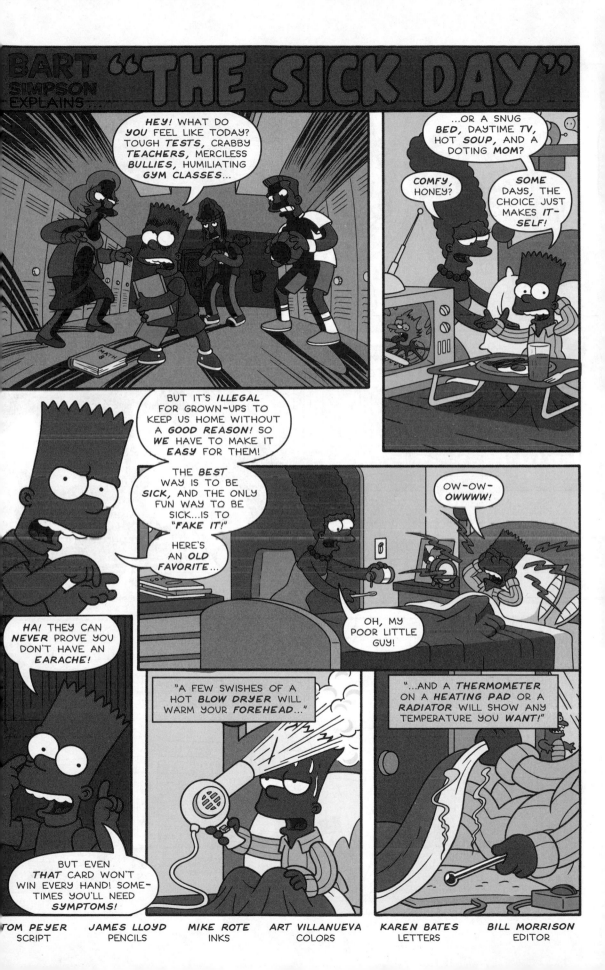

BART SIMPSON EXPLAINS... "THE SICK DAY"

HEY! WHAT DO *YOU* FEEL LIKE TODAY? TOUGH *TESTS,* CRABBY *TEACHERS,* MERCILESS *BULLIES,* HUMILIATING *GYM CLASSES...*

...OR A SNUG *BED,* DAYTIME *TV,* HOT *SOUP,* AND A DOTING *MOM?*

COMFY, HONEY?

SOME DAYS, THE CHOICE JUST MAKES *IT-SELF!*

BUT IT'S *ILLEGAL* FOR GROWN-UPS TO KEEP US HOME WITHOUT A *GOOD REASON!* SO *WE* HAVE TO MAKE IT *EASY* FOR THEM!

THE *BEST* WAY IS TO BE *SICK,* AND THE ONLY FUN WAY TO BE SICK...IS TO *"FAKE IT!"*

HERE'S AN *OLD FAVORITE...*

OW-OW-OWWWW!

HA! THEY CAN *NEVER* PROVE YOU DON'T HAVE AN *EARACHE!*

OH, MY POOR LITTLE GUY!

"A FEW SWISHES OF A HOT *BLOW DRYER* WILL WARM YOUR *FOREHEAD...*"

"...AND A *THERMOMETER* ON A *HEATING PAD* OR A *RADIATOR* WILL SHOW ANY TEMPERATURE YOU *WANT!*"

BUT EVEN *THAT* CARD WON'T WIN EVERY HAND! SOME-TIMES YOU'LL NEED *SYMPTOMS!*

TOM PEYER
SCRIPT

JAMES LLOYD
PENCILS

MIKE ROTE
INKS

ART VILLANUEVA
COLORS

KAREN BATES
LETTERS

BILL MORRISON
EDITOR

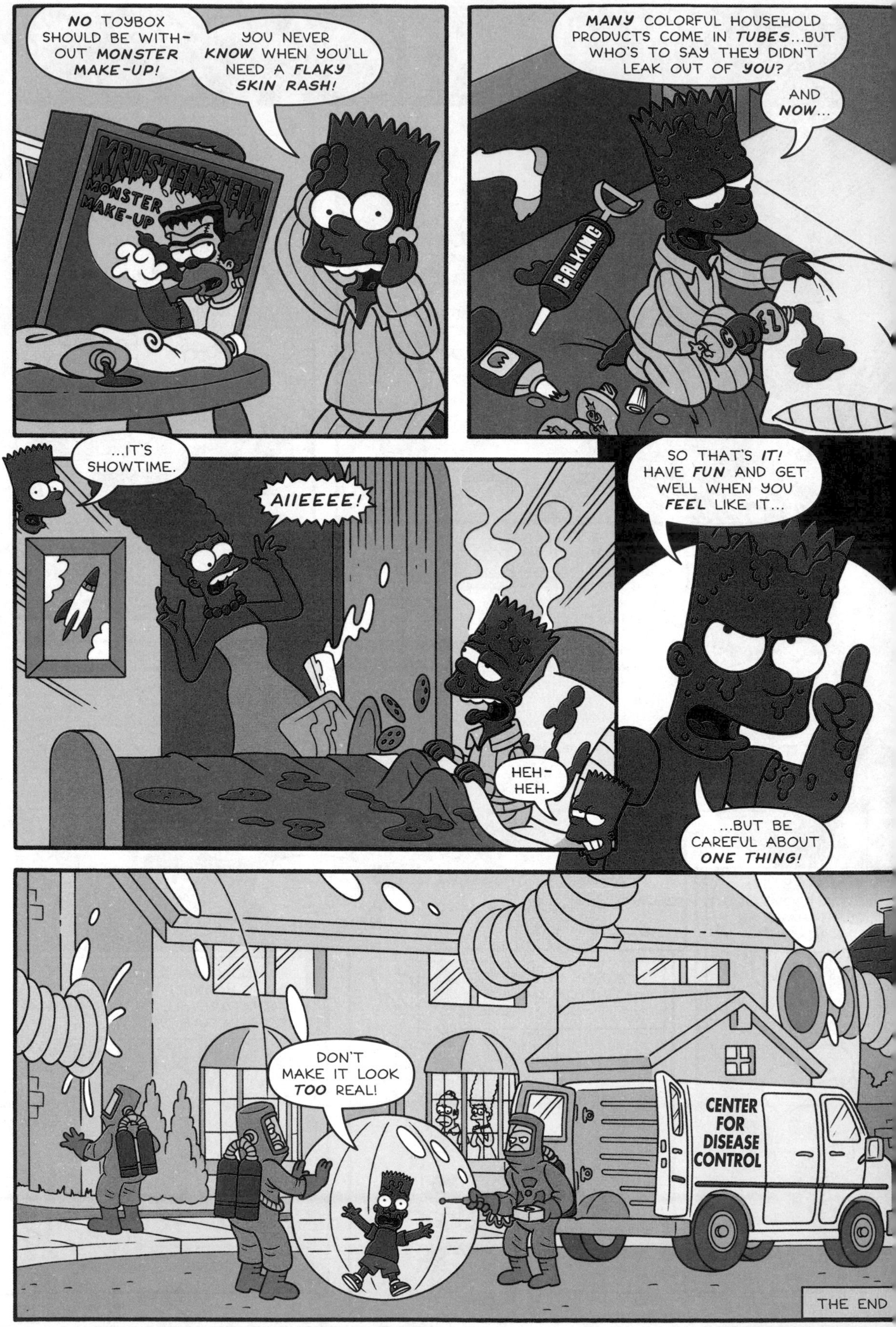
NO TOYBOX SHOULD BE WITH-OUT MONSTER MAKE-UP!
YOU NEVER KNOW WHEN YOU'LL NEED A FLAKY SKIN RASH!
KRUSTENSTEIN MONSTER MAKE-UP
MANY COLORFUL HOUSEHOLD PRODUCTS COME IN TUBES...BUT WHO'S TO SAY THEY DIDN'T LEAK OUT OF YOU?
AND NOW...
CALKING
...IT'S SHOWTIME.
AIIEEEE!
HEH-HEH.
SO THAT'S IT! HAVE FUN AND GET WELL WHEN YOU FEEL LIKE IT...
...BUT BE CAREFUL ABOUT ONE THING!
DON'T MAKE IT LOOK TOO REAL!
CENTER FOR DISEASE CONTROL
THE END

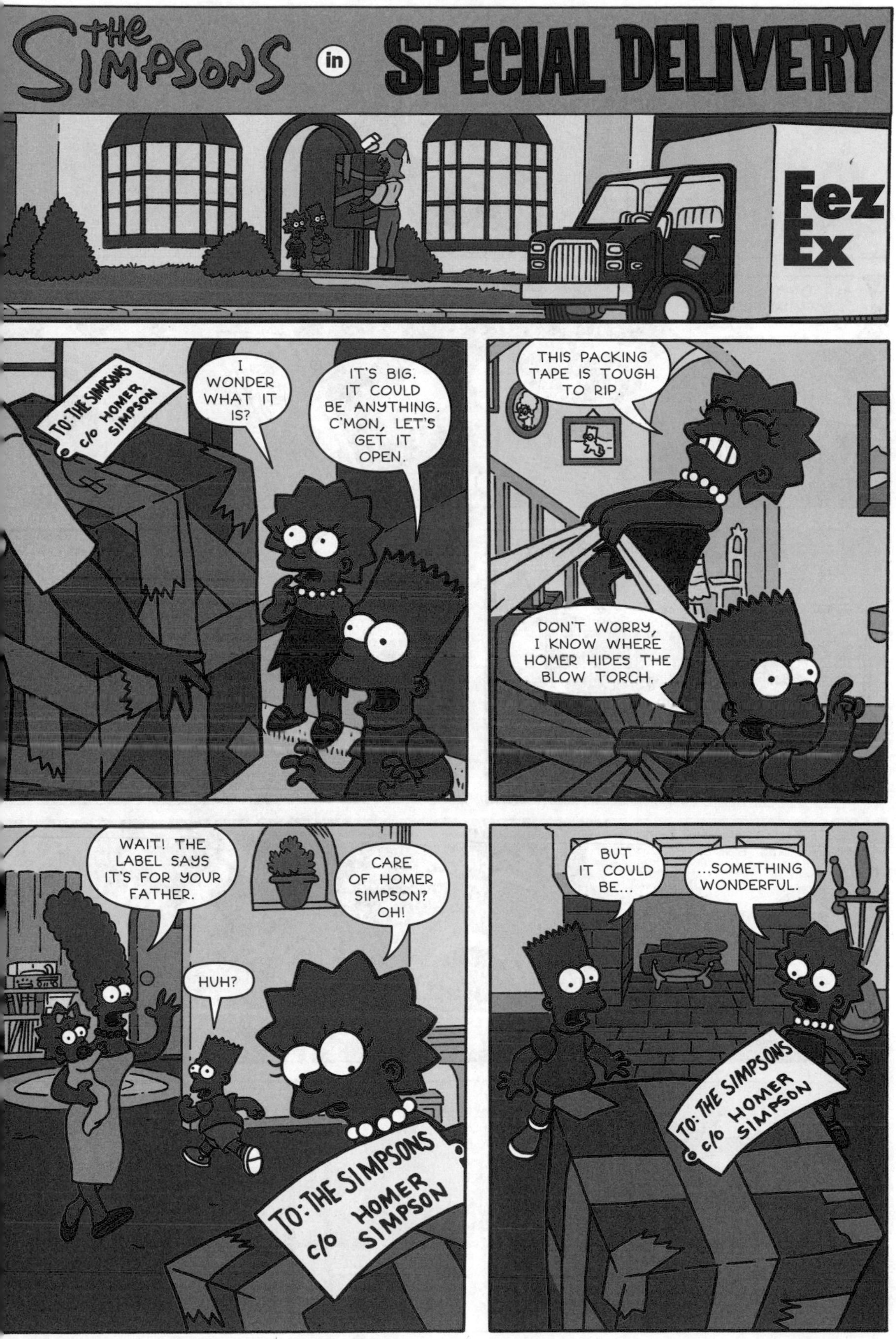

THE SIMPSONS in SPECIAL DELIVERY
Fez Ex
TO: THE SIMPSONS c/o HOMER SIMPSON
I WONDER WHAT IT IS?
IT'S BIG. IT COULD BE ANYTHING. C'MON, LET'S GET IT OPEN.
THIS PACKING TAPE IS TOUGH TO RIP.
DON'T WORRY, I KNOW WHERE HOMER HIDES THE BLOW TORCH.
WAIT! THE LABEL SAYS IT'S FOR YOUR FATHER.
CARE OF HOMER SIMPSON? OH!
HUH?
TO: THE SIMPSONS c/o HOMER SIMPSON
BUT IT COULD BE...
...SOMETHING WONDERFUL.
TO: THE SIMPSONS c/o HOMER SIMPSON

AMES BATES SCRIPT | JOHN DELANEY PENCILS | HOWARD SHUM INKS | ART VILLANUEVA COLORS | KAREN BATES LETTERS | BILL MORRISON EDITOR

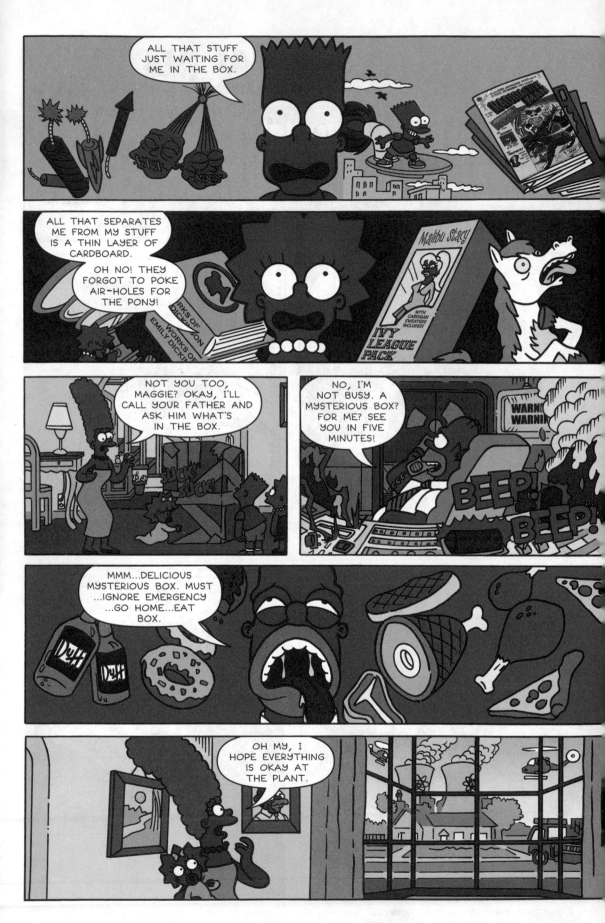

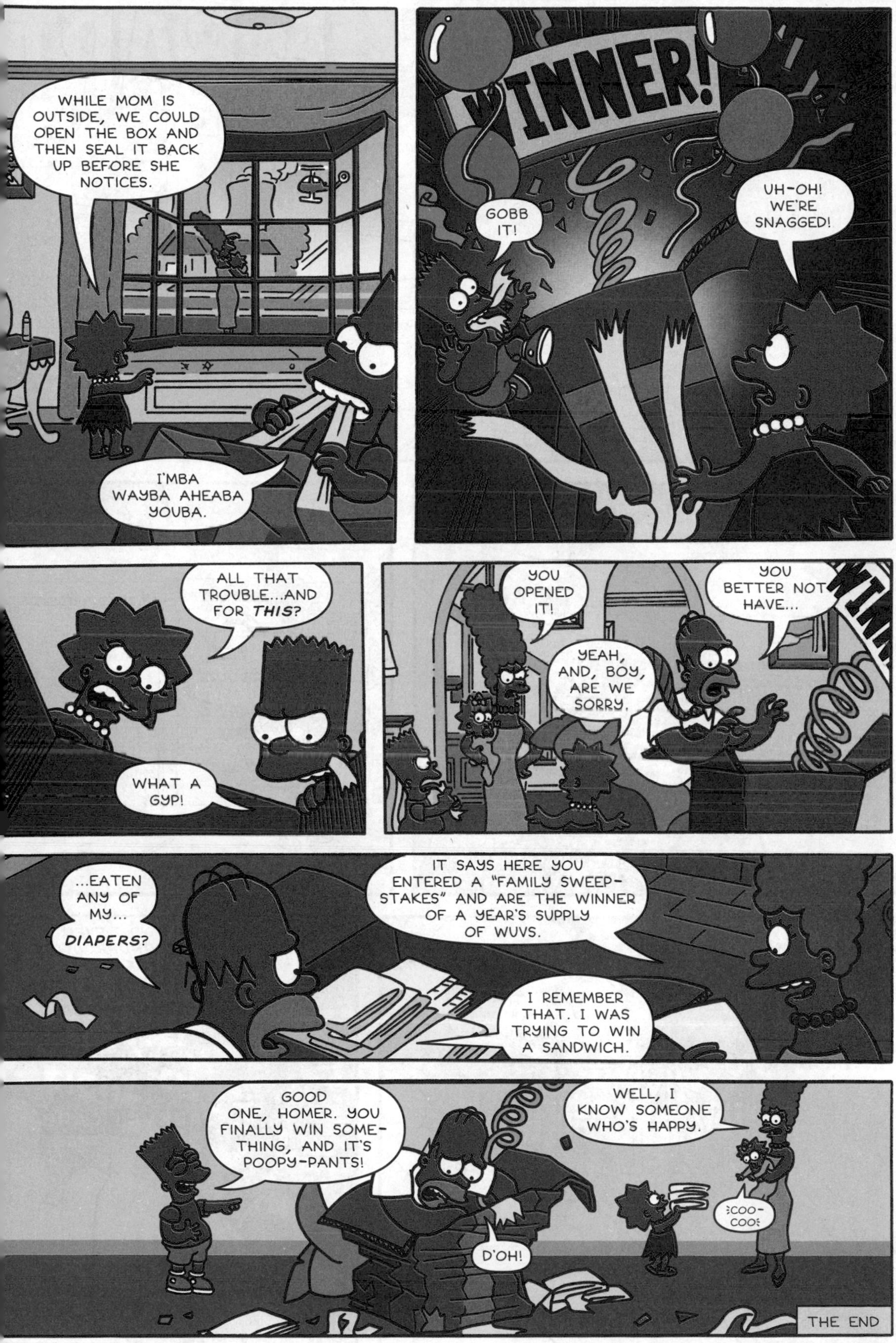
WHILE MOM IS OUTSIDE, WE COULD OPEN THE BOX AND THEN SEAL IT BACK UP BEFORE SHE NOTICES.
I'MBA WAYBA AHEABA YOUBA.
WINNER!
GOBB IT!
UH-OH! WE'RE SNAGGED!
ALL THAT TROUBLE...AND FOR THIS?
WHAT A GYP!
YOU OPENED IT!
YEAH, AND, BOY, ARE WE SORRY.
YOU BETTER NOT HAVE...
...EATEN ANY OF MY... DIAPERS?
IT SAYS HERE YOU ENTERED A "FAMILY SWEEP-STAKES" AND ARE THE WINNER OF A YEAR'S SUPPLY OF WUVS.
I REMEMBER THAT. I WAS TRYING TO WIN A SANDWICH.
GOOD ONE, HOMER. YOU FINALLY WIN SOME-THING, AND IT'S POOPY-PANTS!
WELL, I KNOW SOMEONE WHO'S HAPPY.
COO-COO
D'OH!
THE END

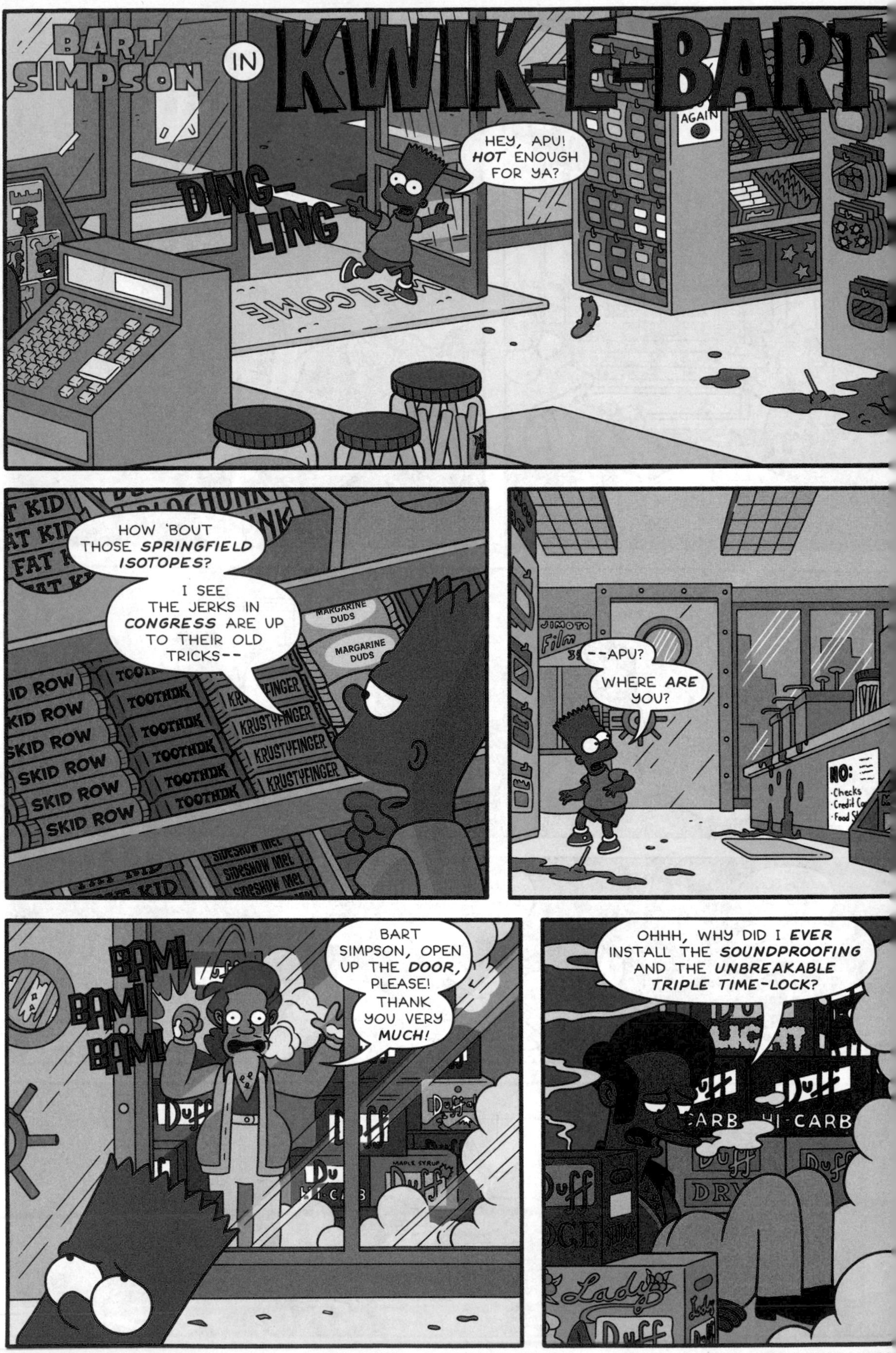
BART SIMPSON IN KWIK-E-BART
DING-LING
HEY, APU! HOT ENOUGH FOR YA?
WELCOME
HOW 'BOUT THOSE SPRINGFIELD ISOTOPES?
I SEE THE JERKS IN CONGRESS ARE UP TO THEIR OLD TRICKS--
--APU?
WHERE ARE YOU?
NO:
-Checks
BAM! BAM! BAM!
BART SIMPSON, OPEN UP THE DOOR, PLEASE! THANK YOU VERY MUCH!
OHHH, WHY DID I EVER INSTALL THE SOUNDPROOFING AND THE UNBREAKABLE TRIPLE TIME-LOCK?

TOM PEYER SCRIPT · JAMES LLOYD PENCILS · MIKE ROTE INKS · NATHAN HAMILL COLORS · KAREN BATES LETTERS · BILL MORRISON EDITOR

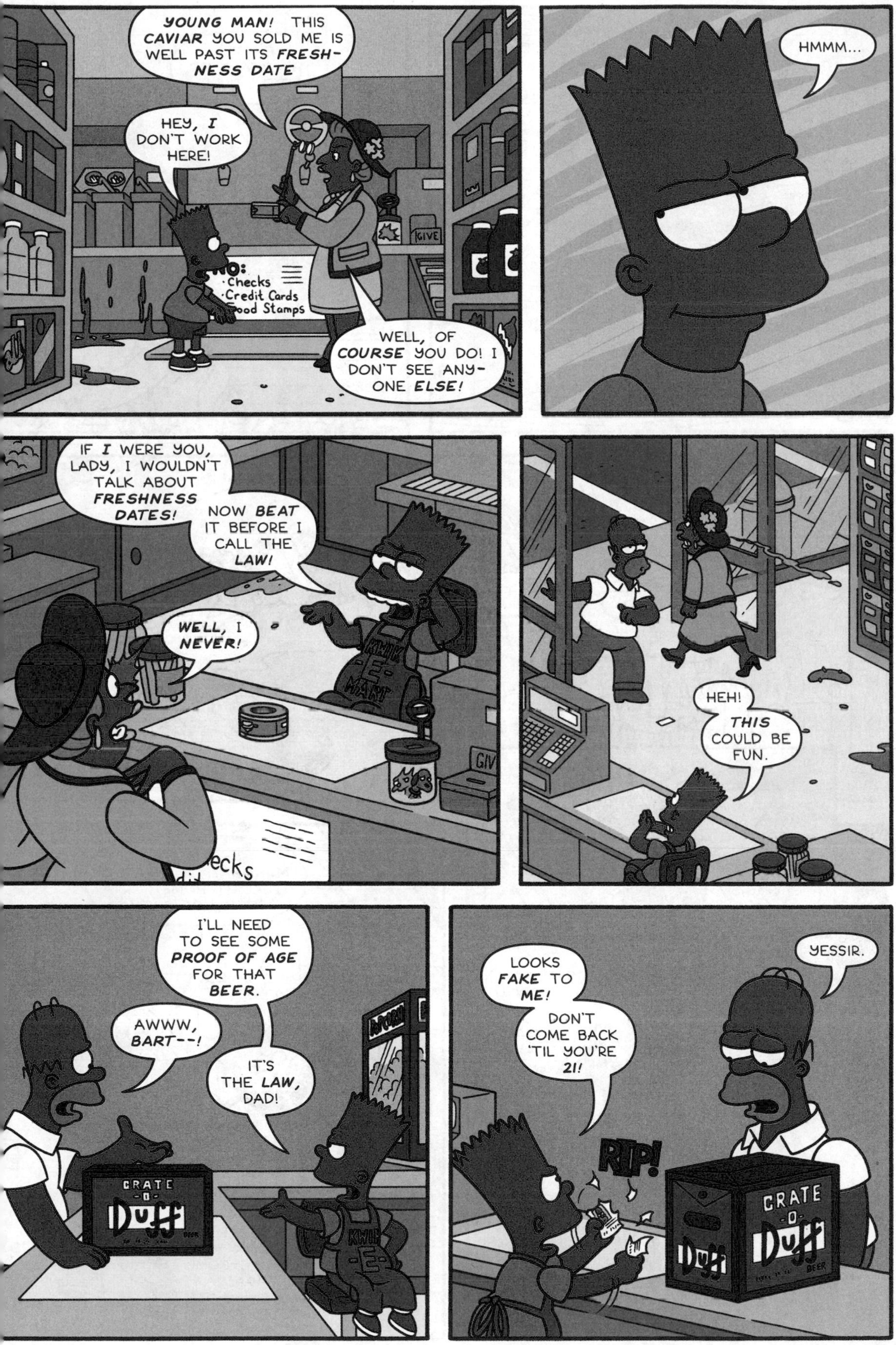

YOUNG MAN! THIS CAVIAR YOU SOLD ME IS WELL PAST ITS FRESHNESS DATE
HEY, I DON'T WORK HERE!
·Checks
·Credit Cards
Food Stamps
GIVE
WELL, OF COURSE YOU DO! I DON'T SEE ANYONE ELSE!
HMMM...
IF I WERE YOU, LADY, I WOULDN'T TALK ABOUT FRESHNESS DATES!
NOW BEAT IT BEFORE I CALL THE LAW!
WELL, I NEVER!
KWIK-E-MART
HEH! THIS COULD BE FUN.
I'LL NEED TO SEE SOME PROOF OF AGE FOR THAT BEER.
AWWW, BART--!
IT'S THE LAW, DAD!
CRATE -O- Duff
LOOKS FAKE TO ME!
DON'T COME BACK 'TIL YOU'RE 21!
YESSIR.
RIP!
CRATE -O- Duff BEER

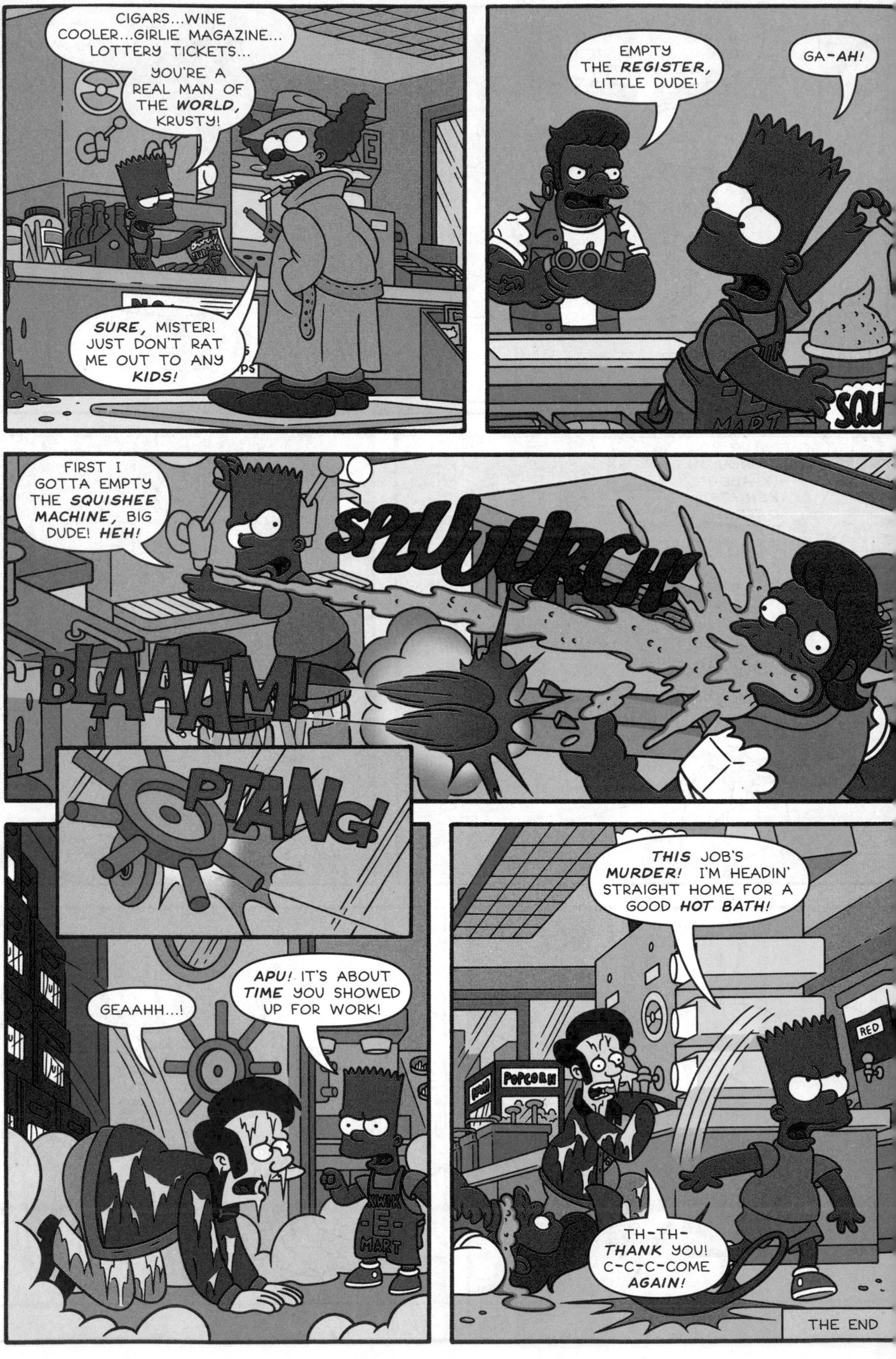
CIGARS...WINE COOLER...GIRLIE MAGAZINE... LOTTERY TICKETS...
YOU'RE A REAL MAN OF THE WORLD, KRUSTY!
SURE, MISTER! JUST DON'T RAT ME OUT TO ANY KIDS!
EMPTY THE REGISTER, LITTLE DUDE!
GA-AH!
FIRST I GOTTA EMPTY THE SQUISHEE MACHINE, BIG DUDE! HEH!
SPLUUURCH!
BLAAAM!
PTANG!
GEAAHH...!
APU! IT'S ABOUT TIME YOU SHOWED UP FOR WORK!
KWIK-E-MART
THIS JOB'S MURDER! I'M HEADIN' STRAIGHT HOME FOR A GOOD HOT BATH!
POPCORN
RED
TH-TH-THANK YOU! C-C-C-COME AGAIN!
THE END

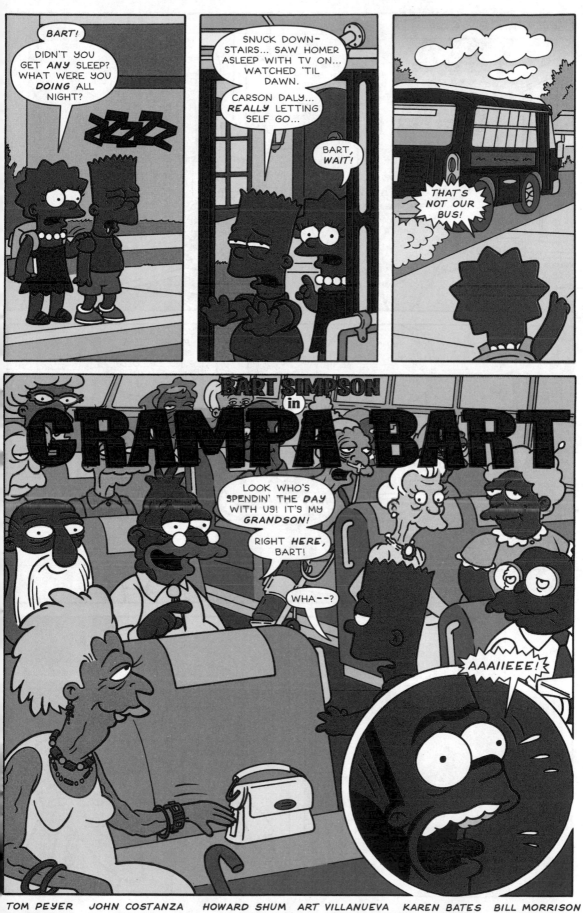

TOM PEYER
SCRIPT

JOHN COSTANZA
PENCILS

HOWARD SHUM
INKS

ART VILLANUEVA
COLORS

KAREN BATES
LETTERS

BILL MORRISON
EDITOR

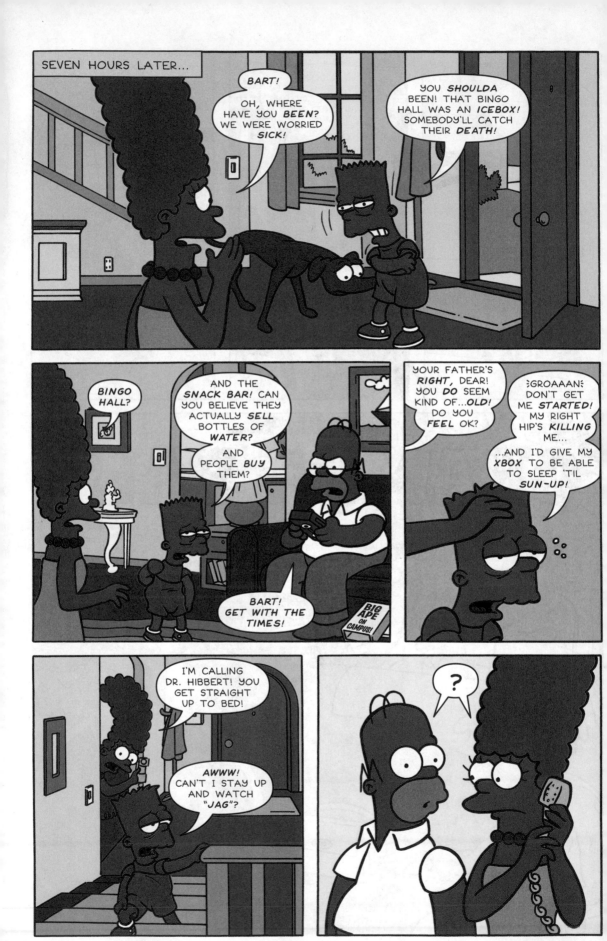

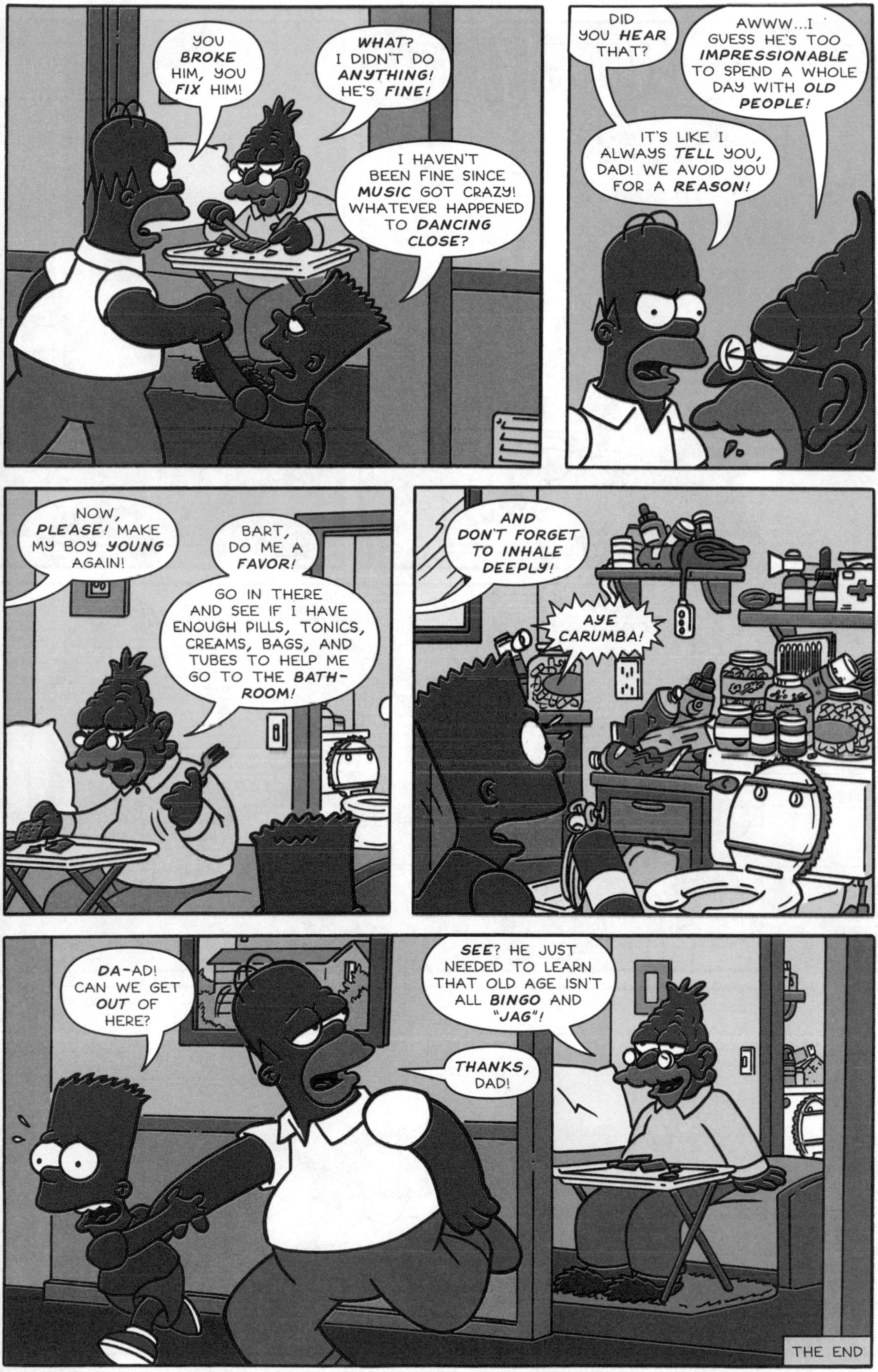
YOU BROKE HIM, YOU FIX HIM!
WHAT? I DIDN'T DO ANYTHING! HE'S FINE!
I HAVEN'T BEEN FINE SINCE MUSIC GOT CRAZY! WHATEVER HAPPENED TO DANCING CLOSE?
DID YOU HEAR THAT?
AWWW...I GUESS HE'S TOO IMPRESSIONABLE TO SPEND A WHOLE DAY WITH OLD PEOPLE!
IT'S LIKE I ALWAYS TELL YOU, DAD! WE AVOID YOU FOR A REASON!
NOW, PLEASE! MAKE MY BOY YOUNG AGAIN!
BART, DO ME A FAVOR!
GO IN THERE AND SEE IF I HAVE ENOUGH PILLS, TONICS, CREAMS, BAGS, AND TUBES TO HELP ME GO TO THE BATH-ROOM!
AND DON'T FORGET TO INHALE DEEPLY!
AYE CARUMBA!
DA-AD! CAN WE GET OUT OF HERE?
SEE? HE JUST NEEDED TO LEARN THAT OLD AGE ISN'T ALL BINGO AND "JAG"!
THANKS, DAD!
THE END

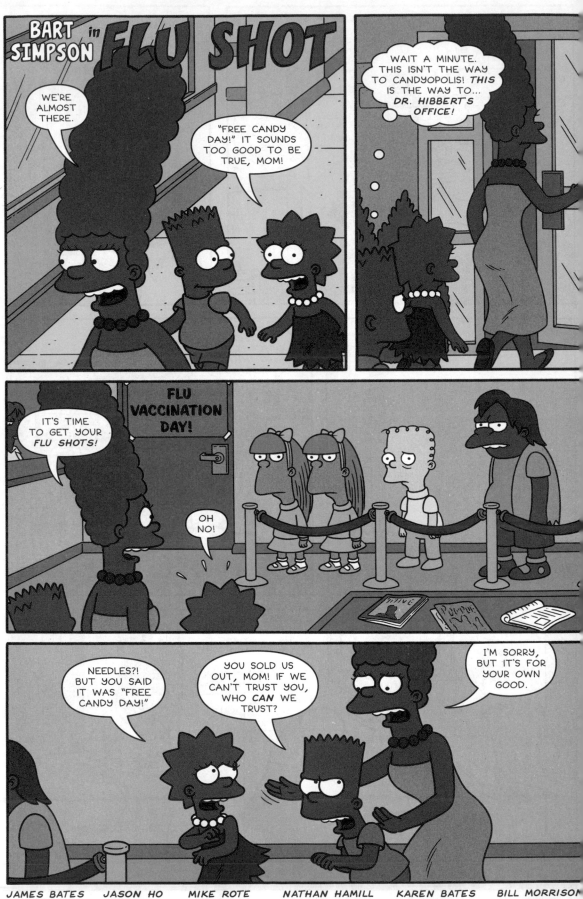

JAMES BATES
SCRIPT

JASON HO
PENCILS

MIKE ROTE
INKS

NATHAN HAMILL
COLORS

KAREN BATES
LETTERS

BILL MORRISON
EDITOR

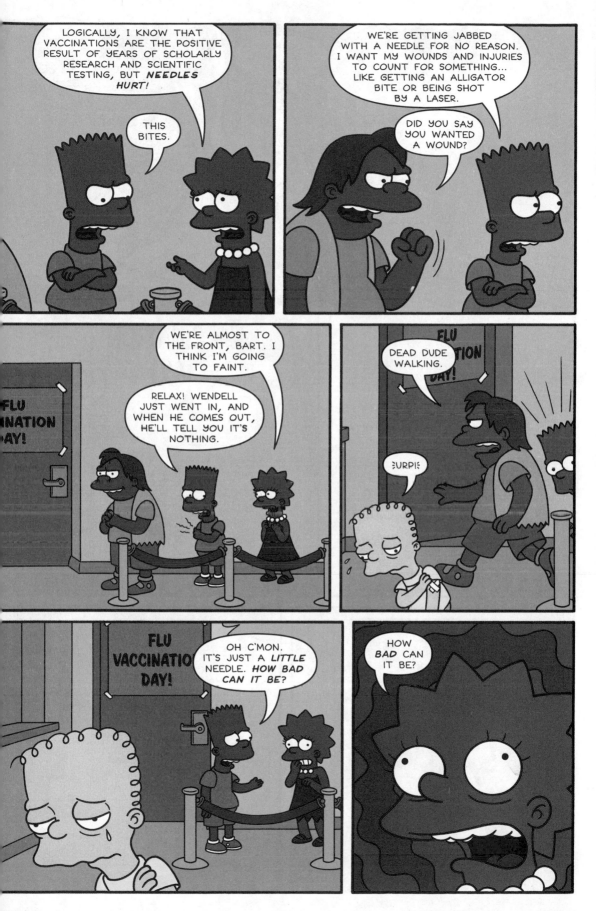

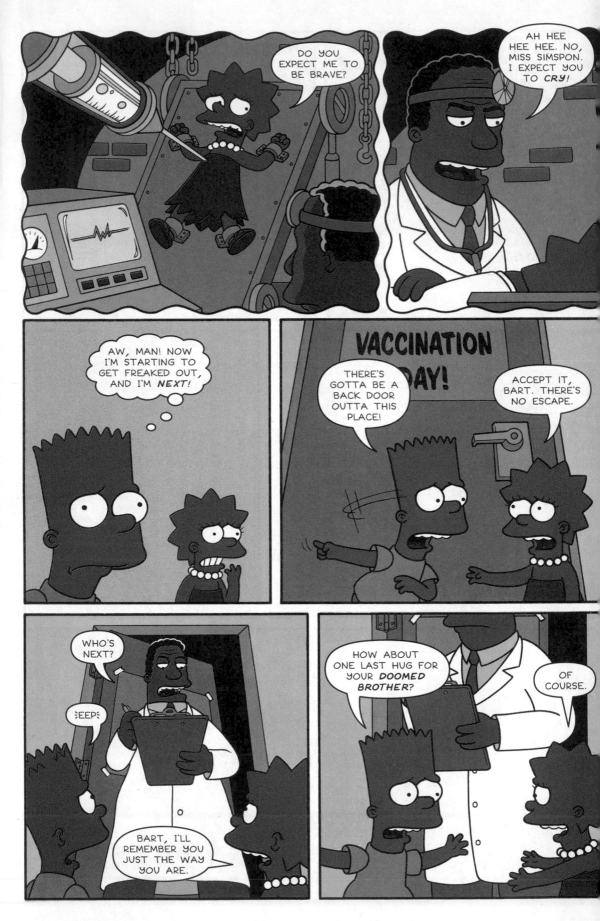

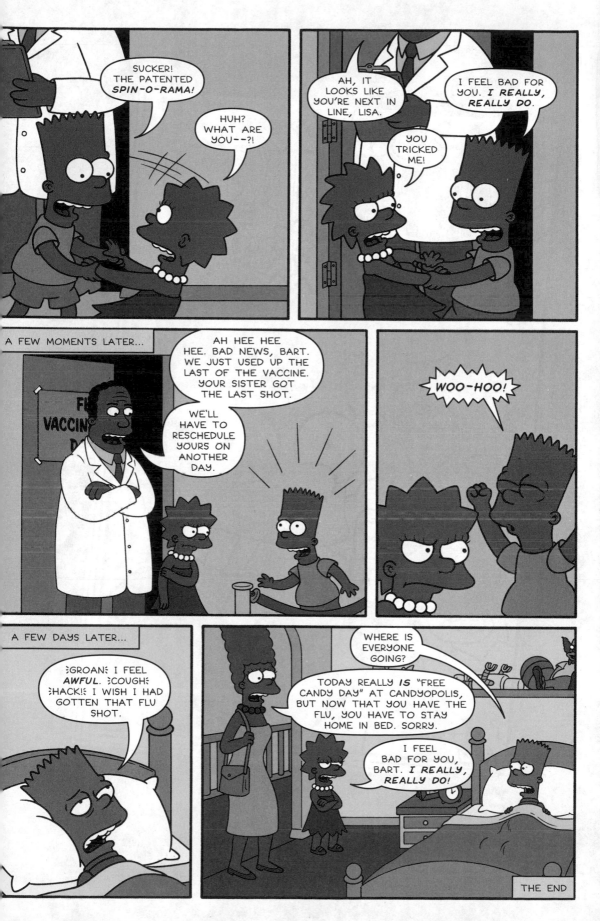

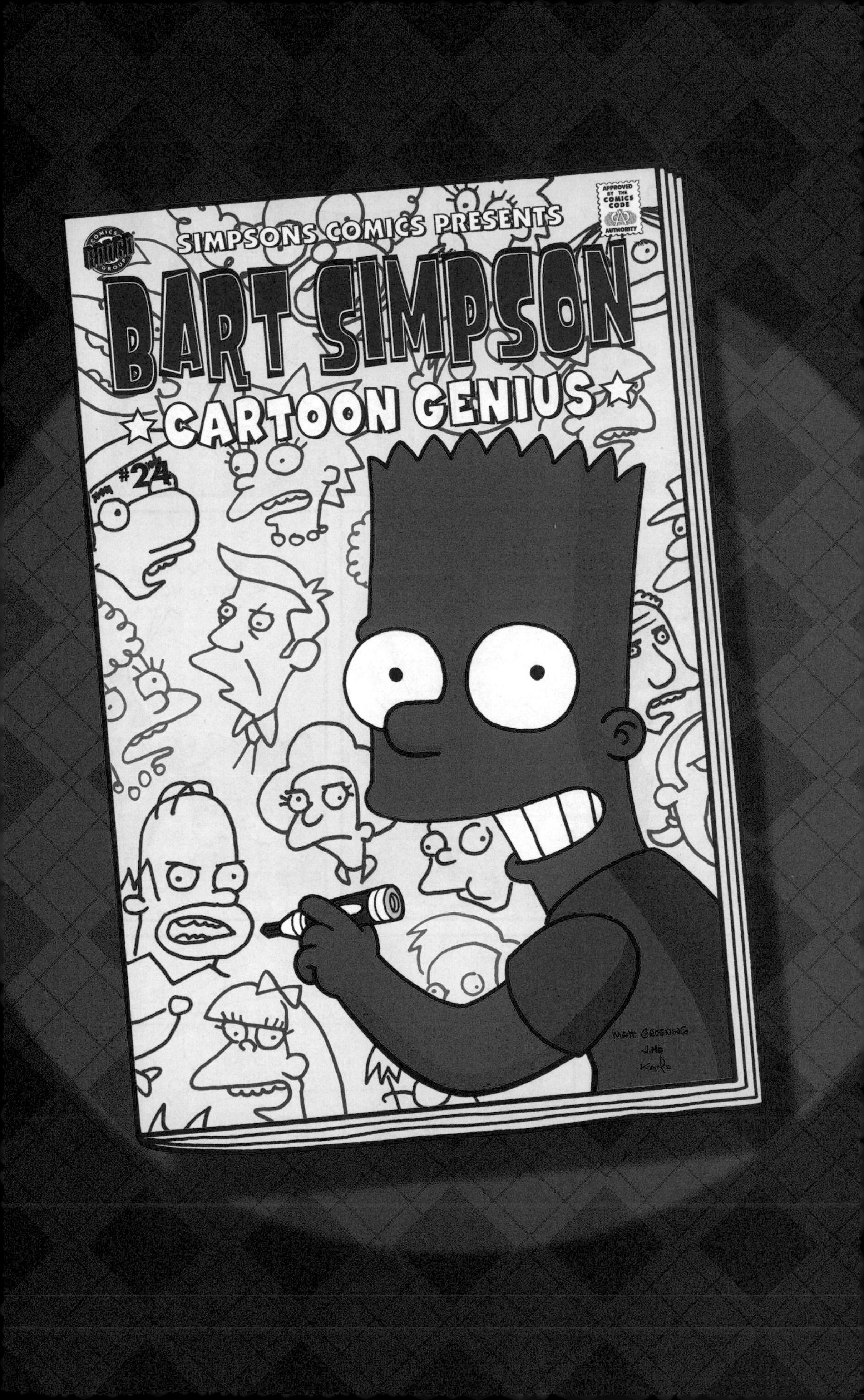
SIMPSONS COMICS PRESENTS
BART SIMPSON
★CARTOON GENIUS★
#24
APPROVED BY THE COMICS CODE AUTHORITY
MATT GROENING
J.HO

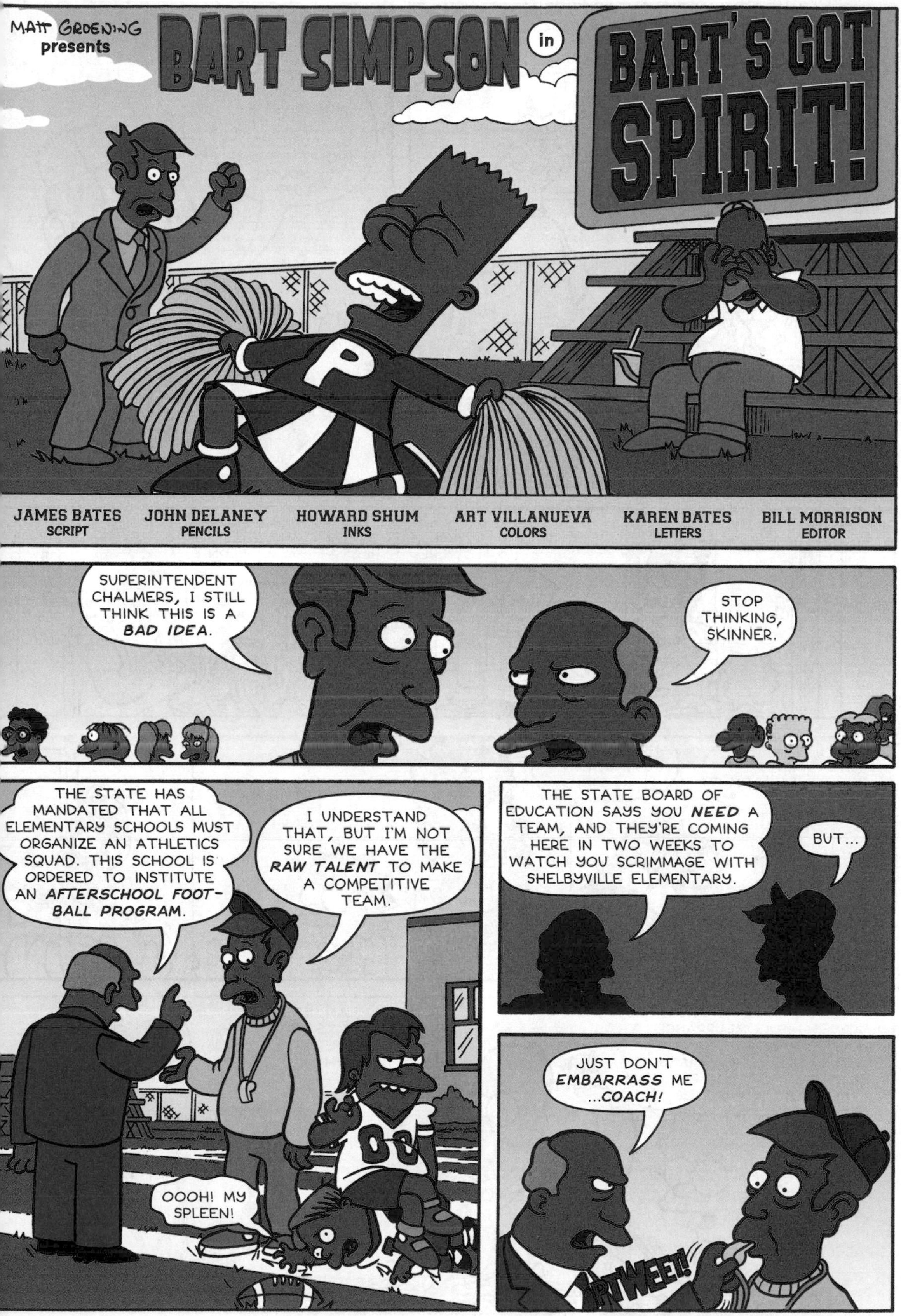
MATT GROENING presents
BART SIMPSON in
BART'S GOT SPIRIT!
P
JAMES BATES SCRIPT
JOHN DELANEY PENCILS
HOWARD SHUM INKS
ART VILLANUEVA COLORS
KAREN BATES LETTERS
BILL MORRISON EDITOR
SUPERINTENDENT CHALMERS, I STILL THINK THIS IS A *BAD IDEA*.
STOP THINKING, SKINNER.
THE STATE HAS MANDATED THAT ALL ELEMENTARY SCHOOLS MUST ORGANIZE AN ATHLETICS SQUAD. THIS SCHOOL IS ORDERED TO INSTITUTE AN *AFTERSCHOOL FOOTBALL PROGRAM*.
I UNDERSTAND THAT, BUT I'M NOT SURE WE HAVE THE *RAW TALENT* TO MAKE A COMPETITIVE TEAM.
OOOH! MY SPLEEN!
THE STATE BOARD OF EDUCATION SAYS YOU *NEED* A TEAM, AND THEY'RE COMING HERE IN TWO WEEKS TO WATCH YOU SCRIMMAGE WITH SHELBYVILLE ELEMENTARY.
BUT...
JUST DON'T *EMBARRASS* ME ...*COACH!*
PTWEET!

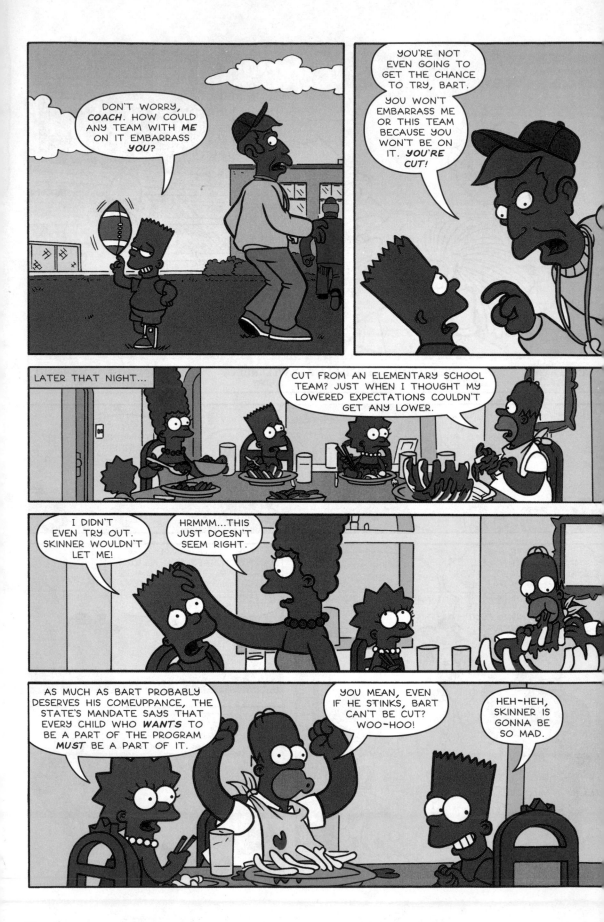

92

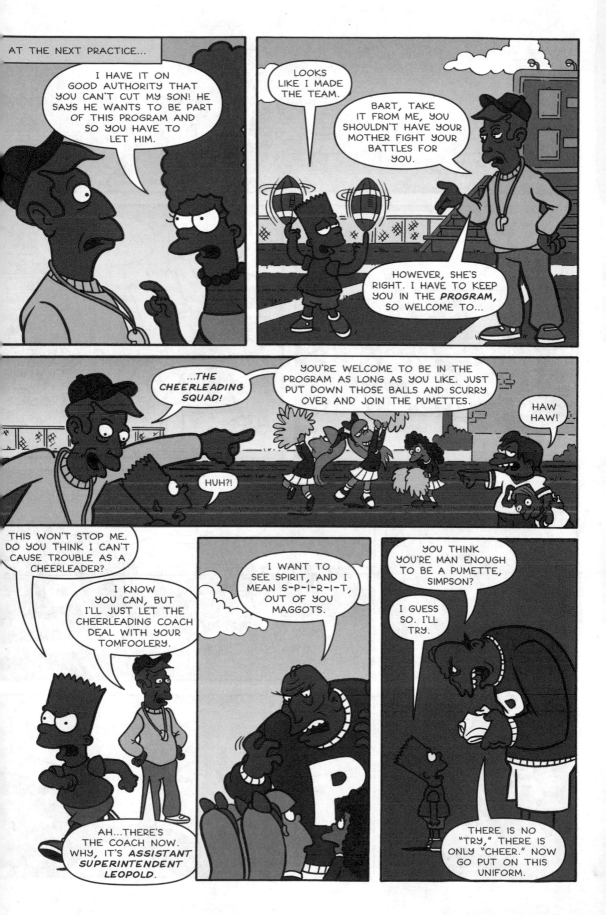

AT THE NEXT PRACTICE...

I HAVE IT ON GOOD AUTHORITY THAT YOU CAN'T CUT MY SON! HE SAYS HE WANTS TO BE PART OF THIS PROGRAM AND SO YOU HAVE TO LET HIM.

LOOKS LIKE I MADE THE TEAM.

BART, TAKE IT FROM ME, YOU SHOULDN'T HAVE YOUR MOTHER FIGHT YOUR BATTLES FOR YOU.

HOWEVER, SHE'S RIGHT. I HAVE TO KEEP YOU IN THE *PROGRAM*, SO WELCOME TO...

...*THE CHEERLEADING SQUAD!*

YOU'RE WELCOME TO BE IN THE PROGRAM AS LONG AS YOU LIKE. JUST PUT DOWN THOSE BALLS AND SCURRY OVER AND JOIN THE PUMETTES.

HAW HAW!

HUH?!

THIS WON'T STOP ME. DO YOU THINK I CAN'T CAUSE TROUBLE AS A CHEERLEADER?

I KNOW YOU CAN, BUT I'LL JUST LET THE CHEERLEADING COACH DEAL WITH YOUR TOMFOOLERY.

AH...THERE'S THE COACH NOW. WHY, IT'S *ASSISTANT SUPERINTENDENT LEOPOLD.*

I WANT TO SEE SPIRIT, AND I MEAN S-P-I-R-I-T, OUT OF YOU MAGGOTS.

YOU THINK YOU'RE MAN ENOUGH TO BE A PUMETTE, SIMPSON?

I GUESS SO. I'LL TRY.

THERE IS NO "TRY," THERE IS ONLY "CHEER." NOW GO PUT ON THIS UNIFORM.

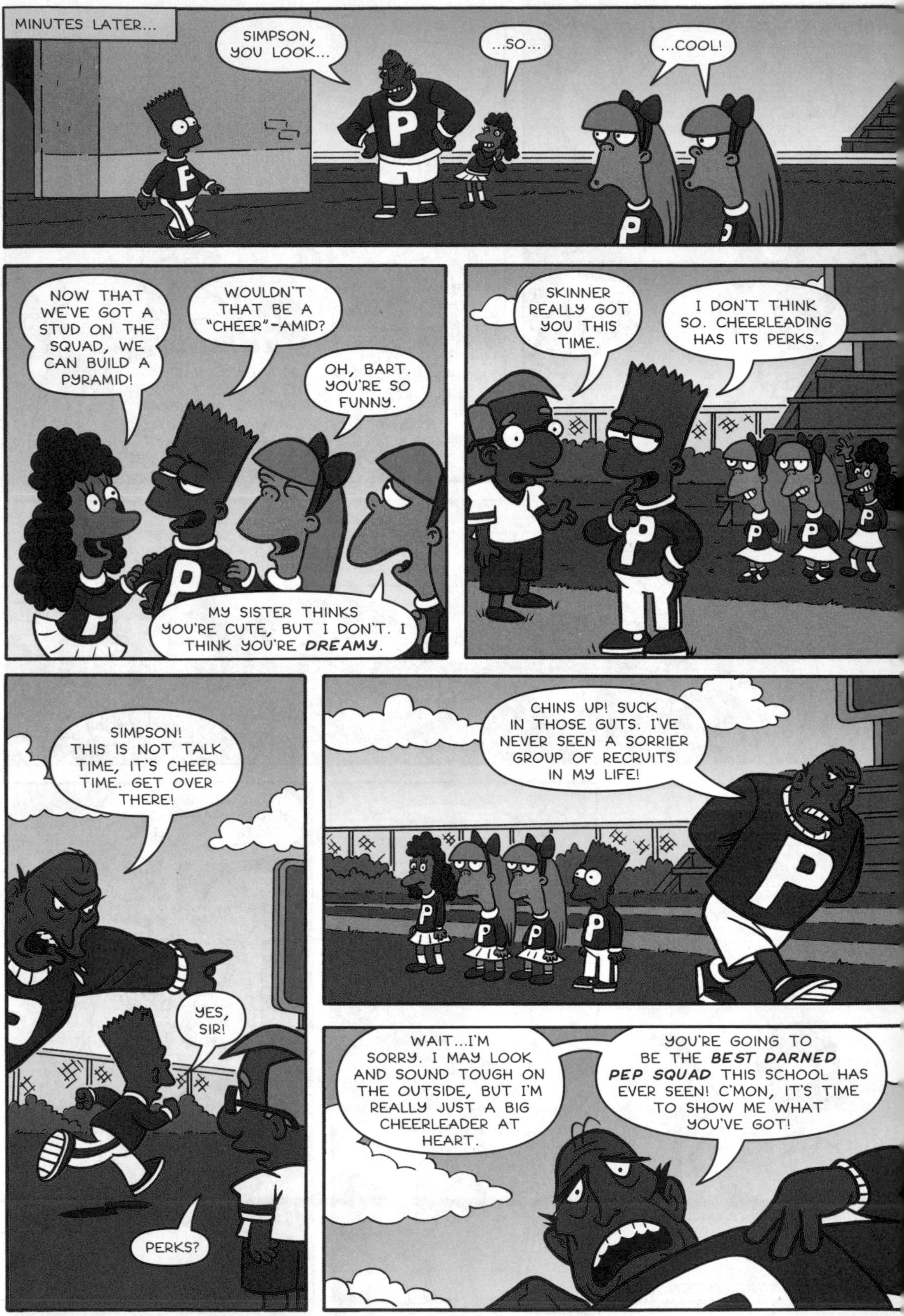
MINUTES LATER...
SIMPSON, YOU LOOK...
...SO...
...COOL!
NOW THAT WE'VE GOT A STUD ON THE SQUAD, WE CAN BUILD A PYRAMID!
WOULDN'T THAT BE A "CHEER"-AMID?
OH, BART. YOU'RE SO FUNNY.
MY SISTER THINKS YOU'RE CUTE, BUT I DON'T. I THINK YOU'RE ***DREAMY***.
SKINNER REALLY GOT YOU THIS TIME.
I DON'T THINK SO. CHEERLEADING HAS ITS PERKS.
SIMPSON! THIS IS NOT TALK TIME, IT'S CHEER TIME. GET OVER THERE!
YES, SIR!
PERKS?
CHINS UP! SUCK IN THOSE GUTS. I'VE NEVER SEEN A SORRIER GROUP OF RECRUITS IN MY LIFE!
WAIT...I'M SORRY. I MAY LOOK AND SOUND TOUGH ON THE OUTSIDE, BUT I'M REALLY JUST A BIG CHEERLEADER AT HEART.
YOU'RE GOING TO BE THE ***BEST DARNED PEP SQUAD*** THIS SCHOOL HAS EVER SEEN! C'MON, IT'S TIME TO SHOW ME WHAT YOU'VE GOT!

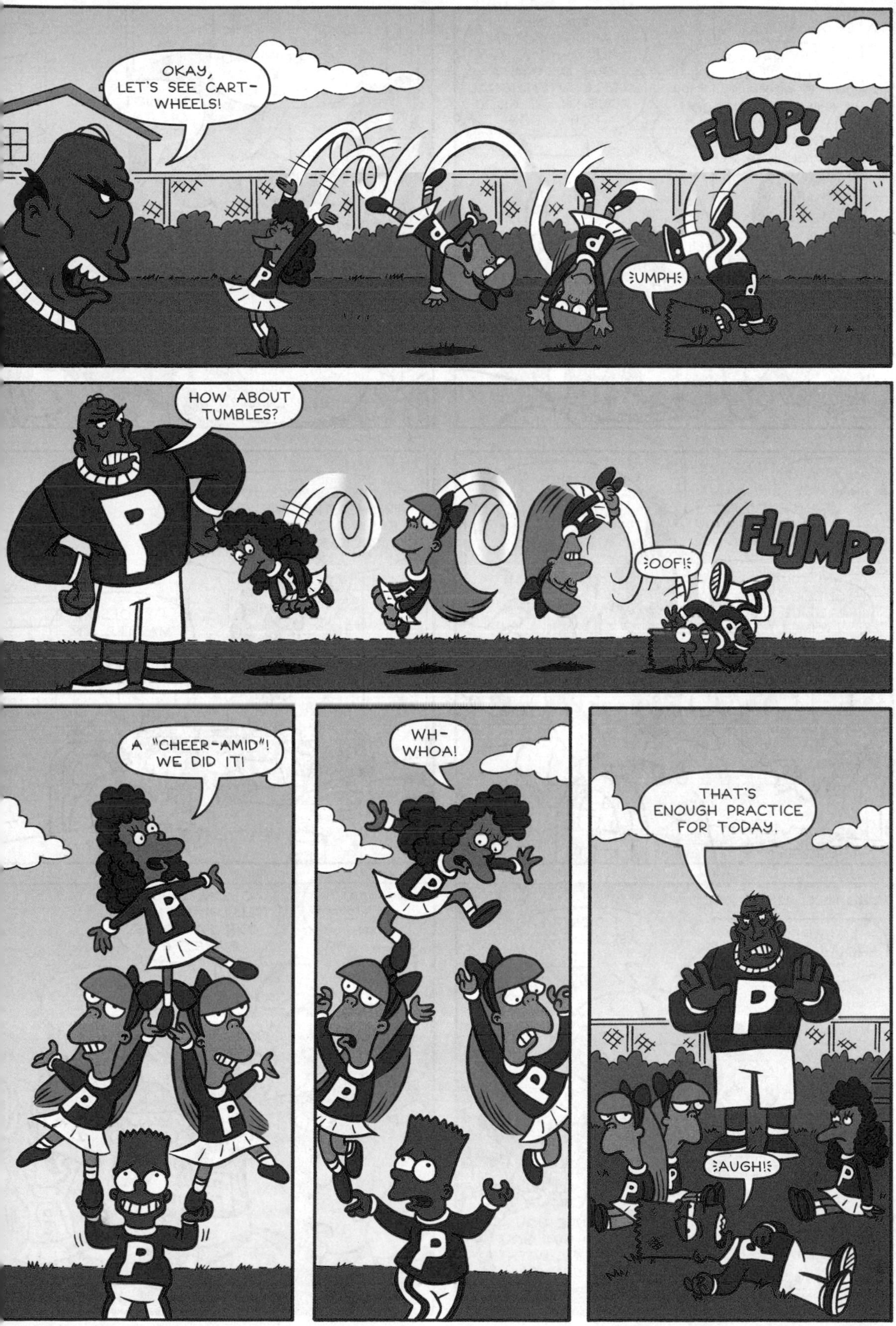
OKAY, LET'S SEE CART-WHEELS!
FLOP!
UMPH
HOW ABOUT TUMBLES?
OOF!
FLUMP!
A "CHEER-AMID"! WE DID IT!
WH-WHOA!
THAT'S ENOUGH PRACTICE FOR TODAY.
AUGH!

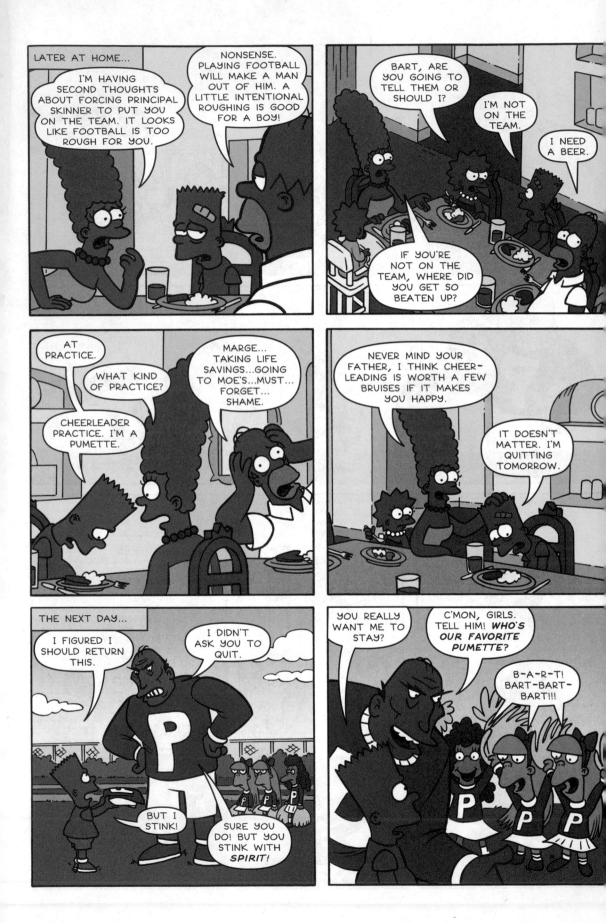

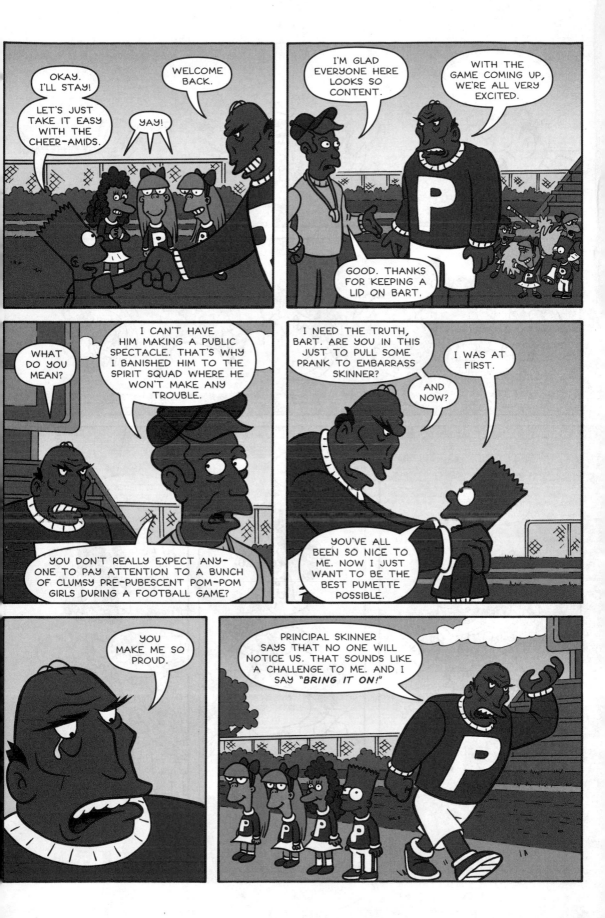

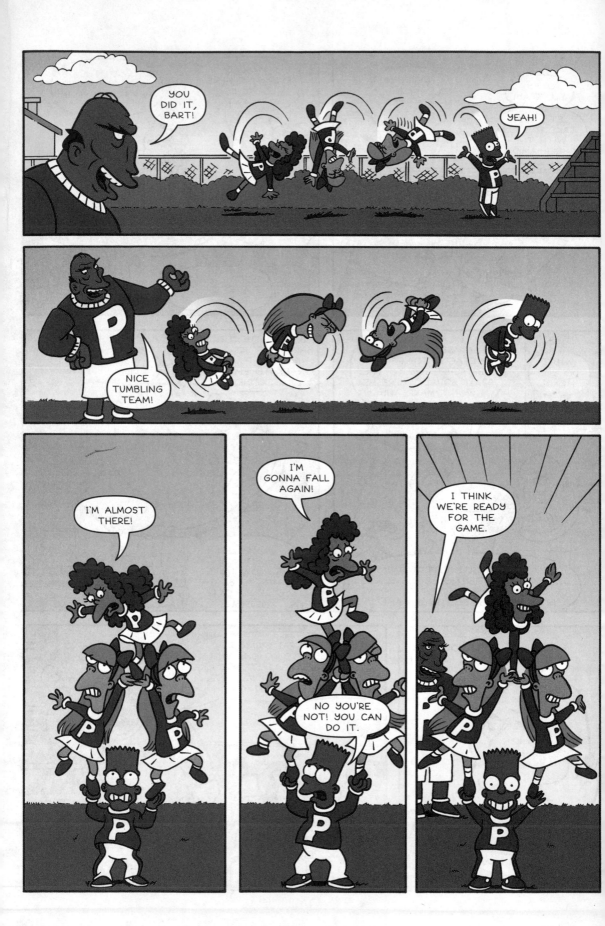

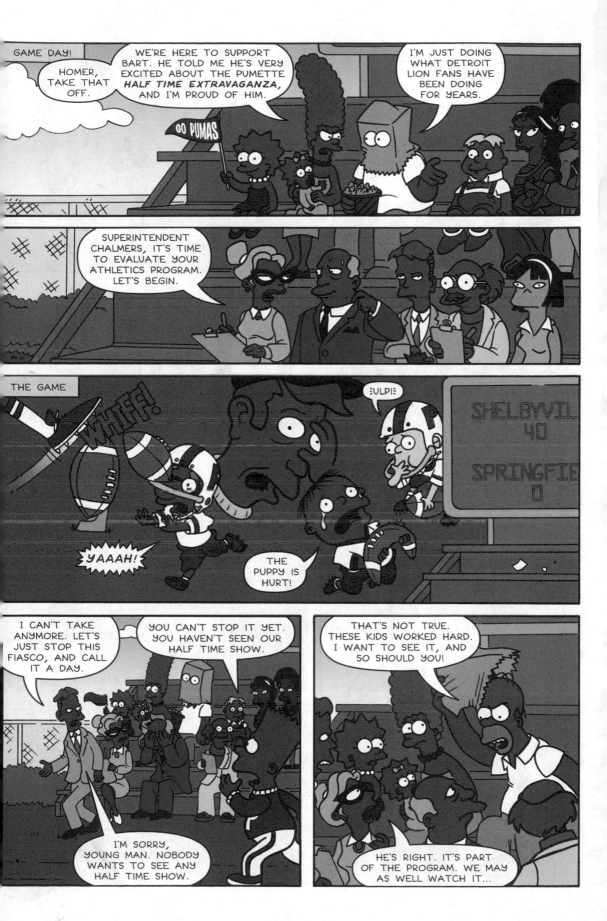

GAME DAY!

HOMER, TAKE THAT OFF.

WE'RE HERE TO SUPPORT BART. HE TOLD ME HE'S VERY EXCITED ABOUT THE PUMETTE *HALF TIME EXTRAVAGANZA*, AND I'M PROUD OF HIM.

I'M JUST DOING WHAT DETROIT LION FANS HAVE BEEN DOING FOR YEARS.

GO PUMAS

SUPERINTENDENT CHALMERS, IT'S TIME TO EVALUATE YOUR ATHLETICS PROGRAM. LET'S BEGIN.

THE GAME

WHTFF!

GULP!

SHELBYVIL 40

SPRINGFIE 0

YAAAH!

THE PUPPY IS HURT!

I CAN'T TAKE ANYMORE. LET'S JUST STOP THIS FIASCO, AND CALL IT A DAY.

YOU CAN'T STOP IT YET. YOU HAVEN'T SEEN OUR HALF TIME SHOW.

I'M SORRY, YOUNG MAN. NOBODY WANTS TO SEE ANY HALF TIME SHOW.

THAT'S NOT TRUE. THESE KIDS WORKED HARD. I WANT TO SEE IT, AND SO SHOULD YOU!

HE'S RIGHT. IT'S PART OF THE PROGRAM. WE MAY AS WELL WATCH IT...

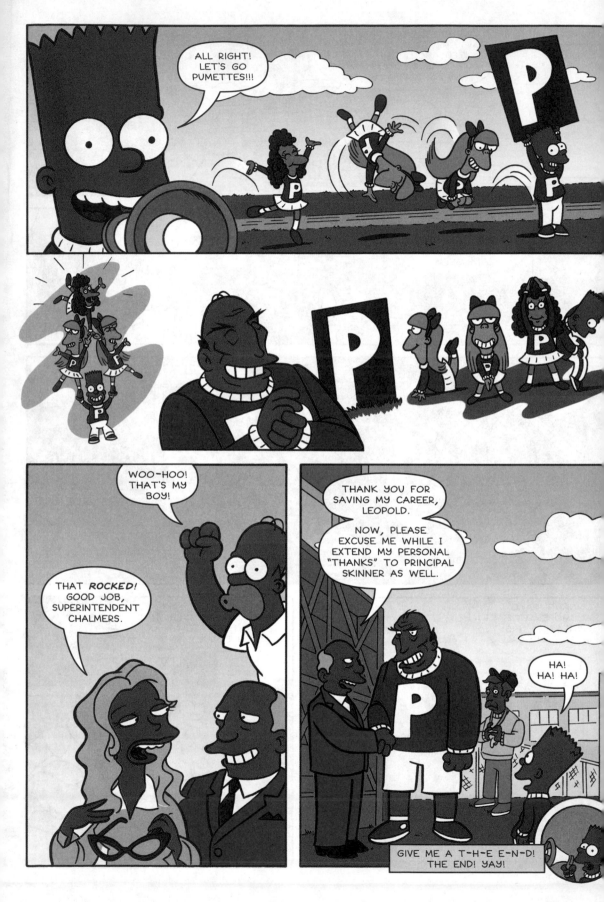

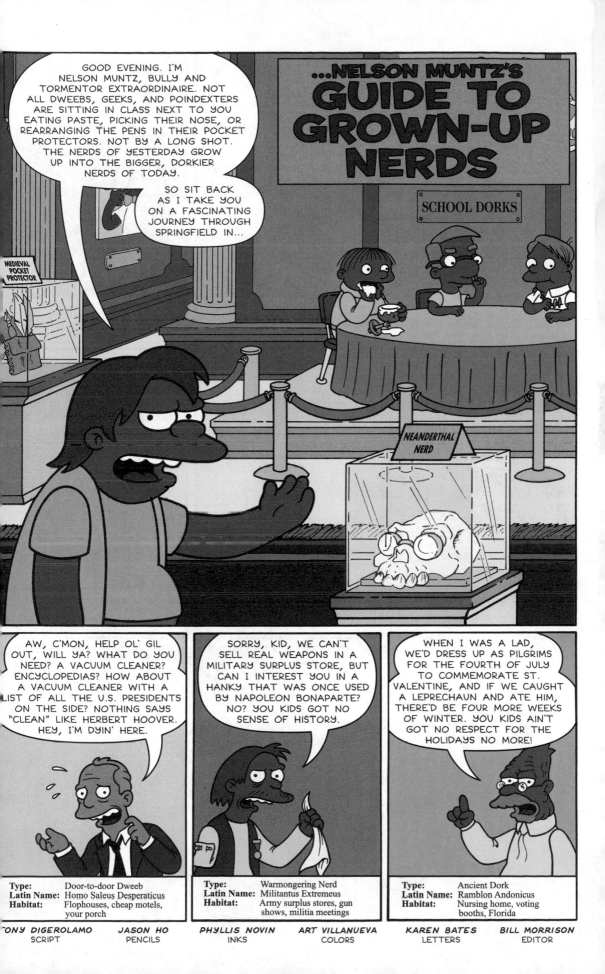

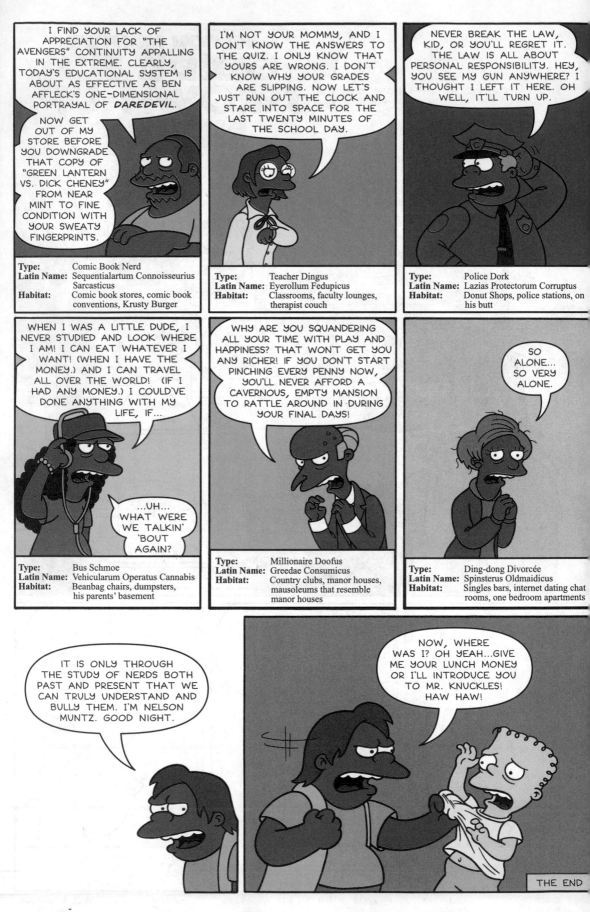

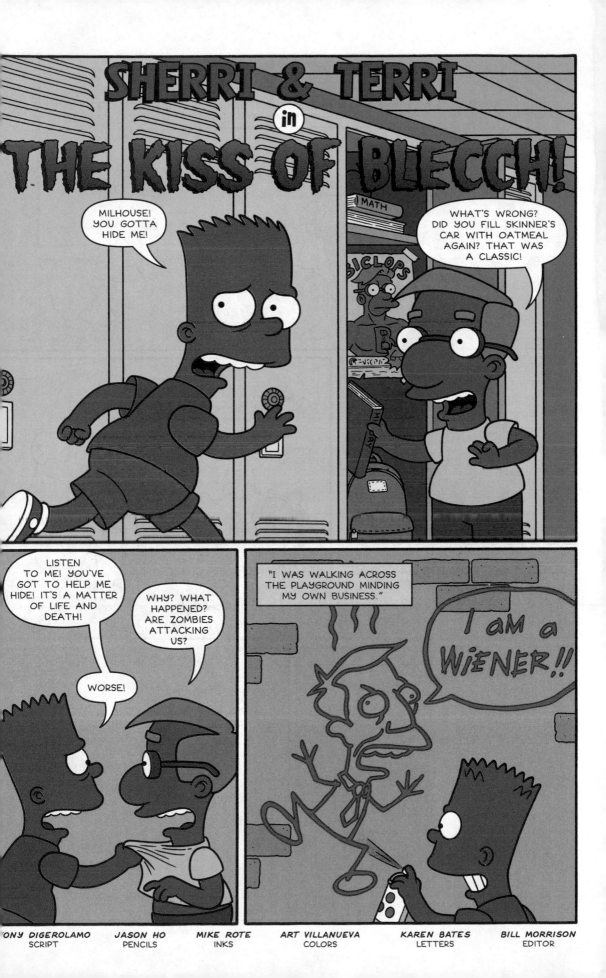

SHERRI & TERRI

in THE KISS OF BLECCH!

MILHOUSE! YOU GOTTA HIDE ME!

WHAT'S WRONG? DID YOU FILL SKINNER'S CAR WITH OATMEAL AGAIN? THAT WAS A CLASSIC!

MATH

BICLOPS

LISTEN TO ME! YOU'VE GOT TO HELP ME HIDE! IT'S A MATTER OF LIFE AND DEATH!

WHY? WHAT HAPPENED? ARE ZOMBIES ATTACKING US?

WORSE!

"I WAS WALKING ACROSS THE PLAYGROUND MINDING MY OWN BUSINESS."

I am a WiENER!!

TONY DIGEROLAMO
SCRIPT

JASON HO
PENCILS

MIKE ROTE
INKS

ART VILLANUEVA
COLORS

KAREN BATES
LETTERS

BILL MORRISON
EDITOR

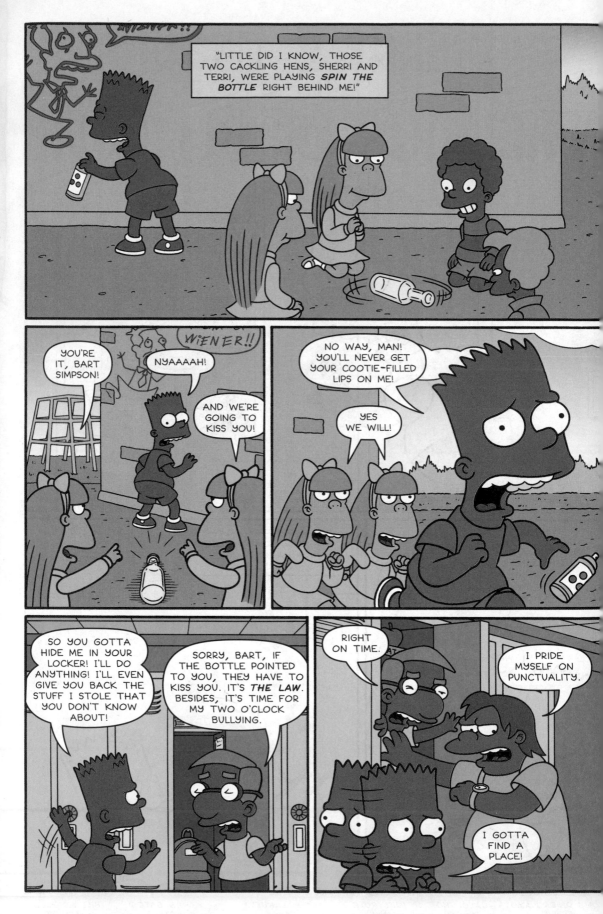

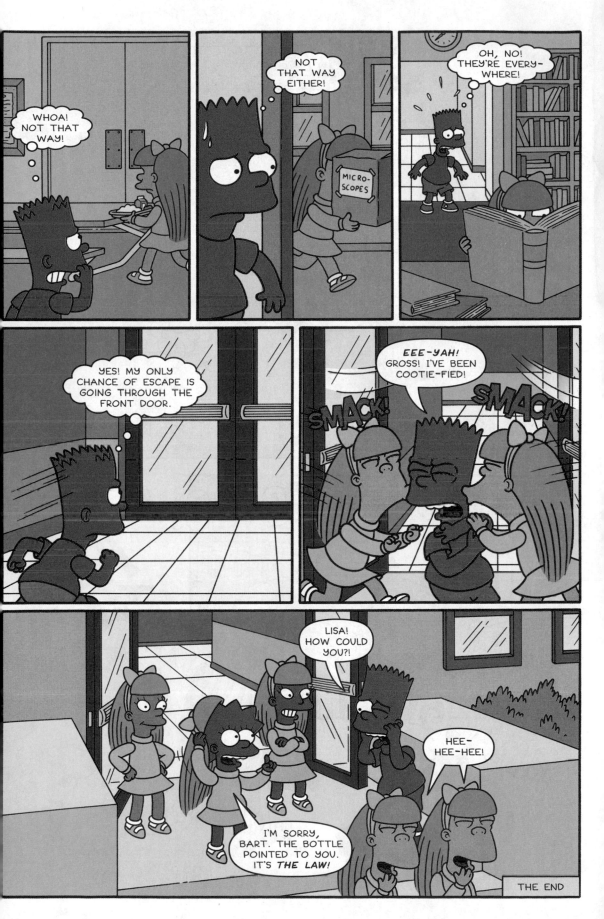

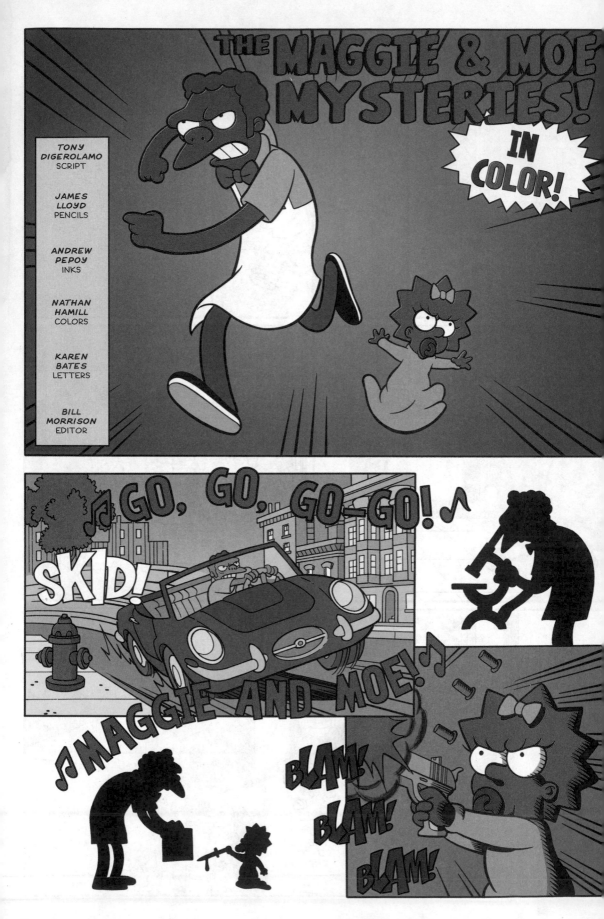

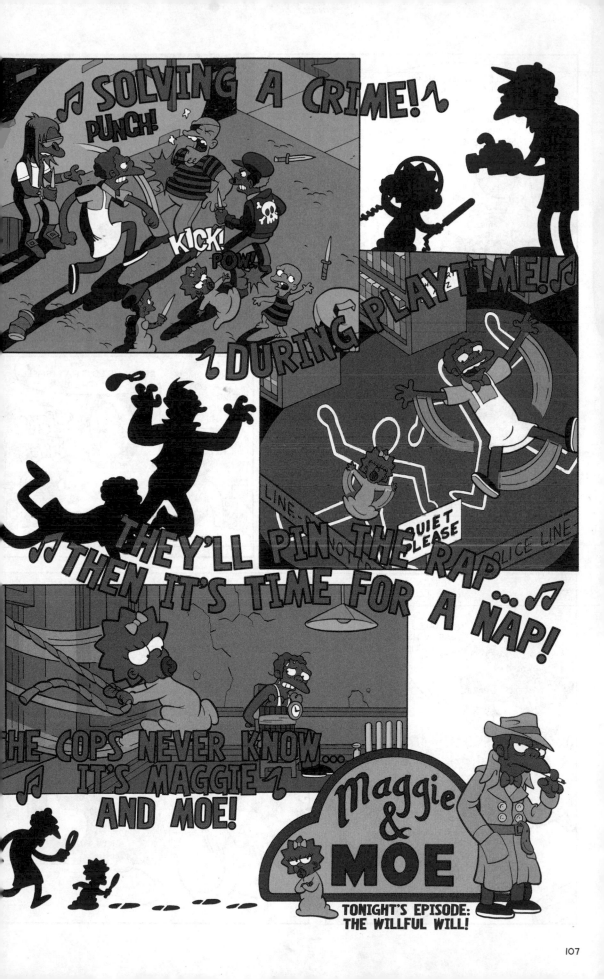

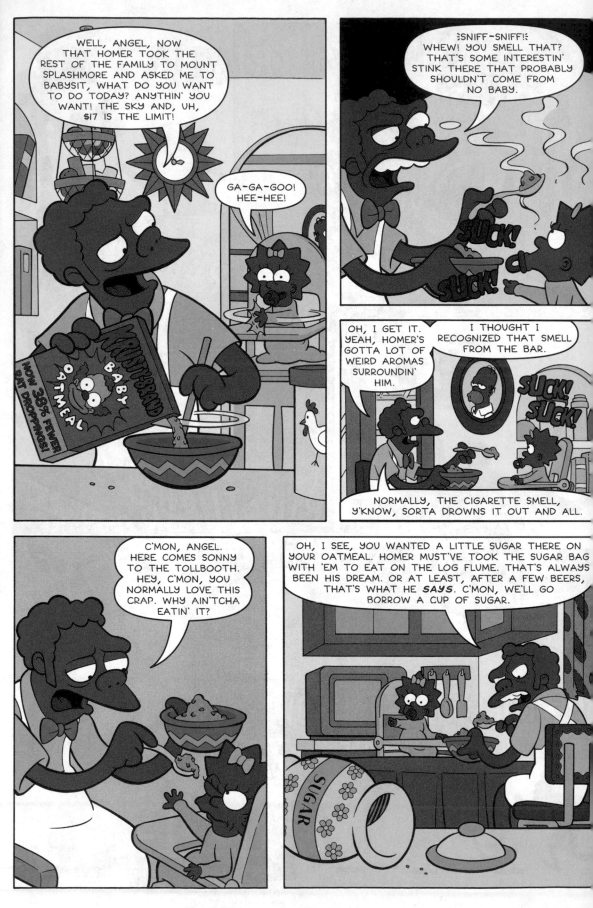

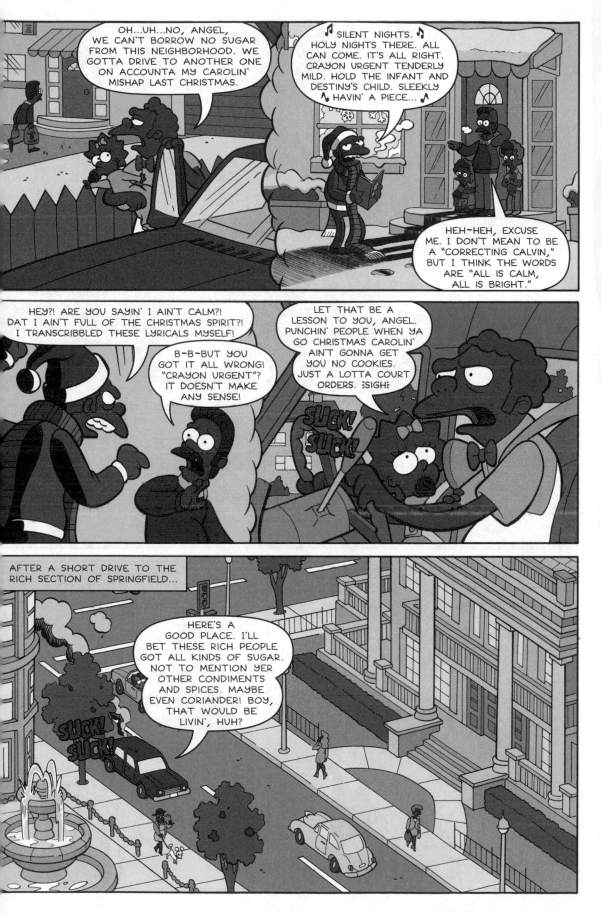

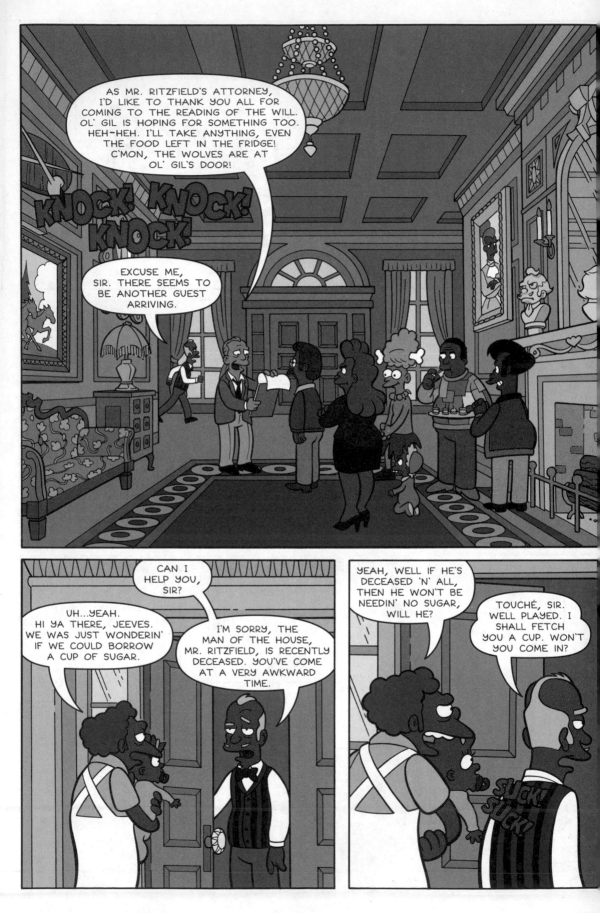

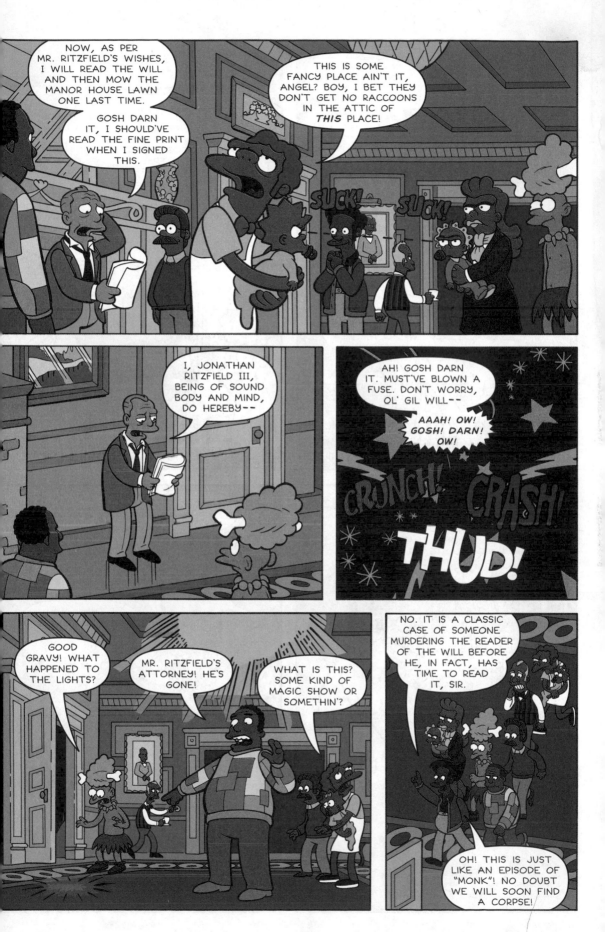

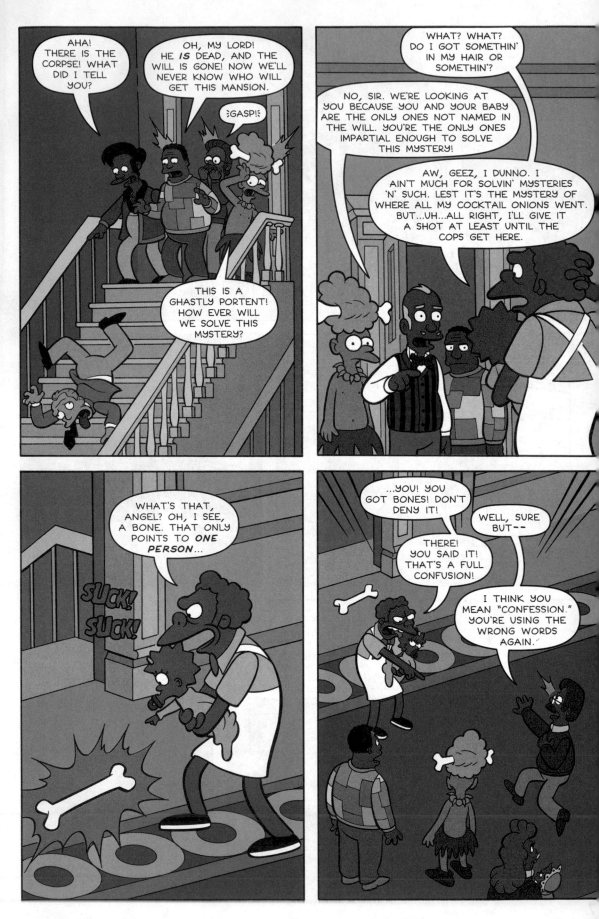

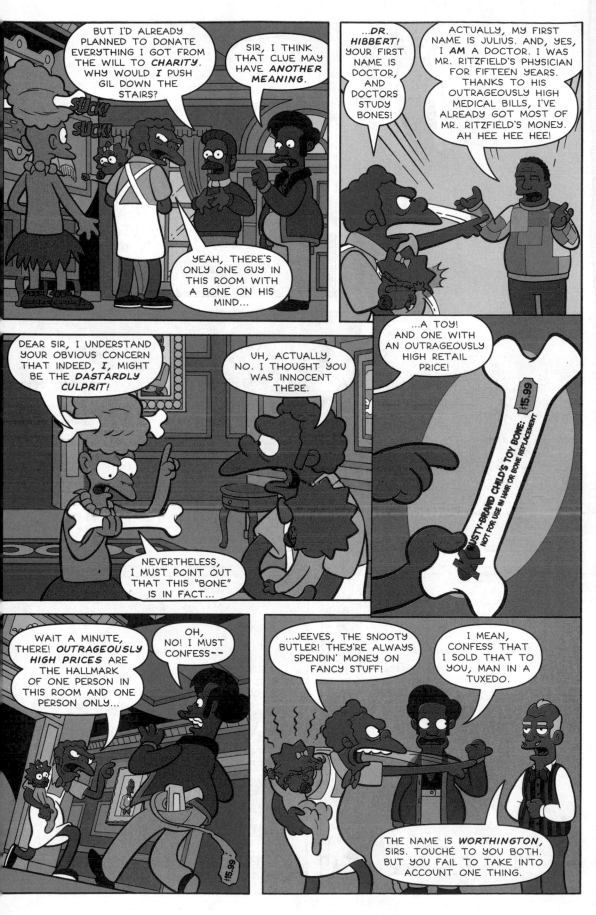

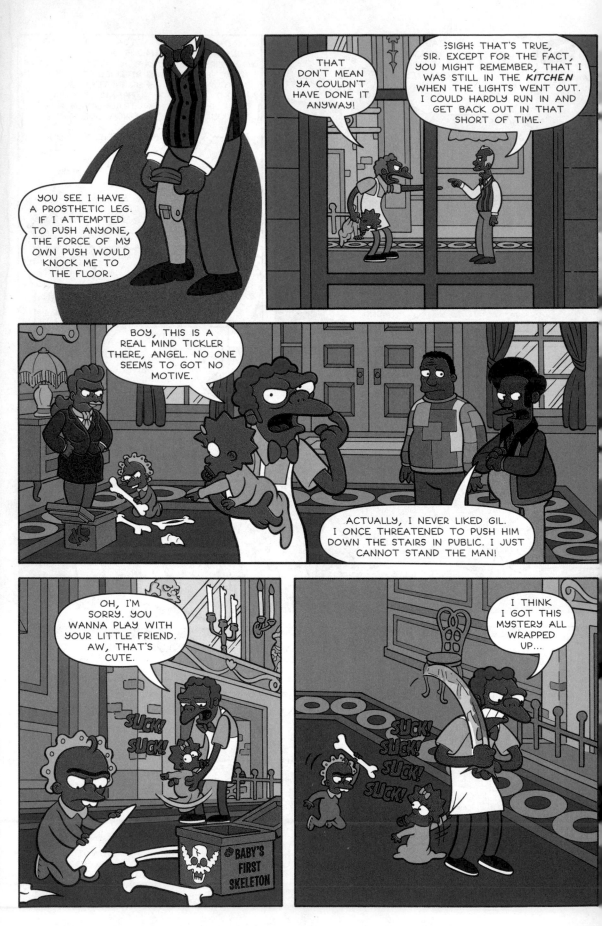

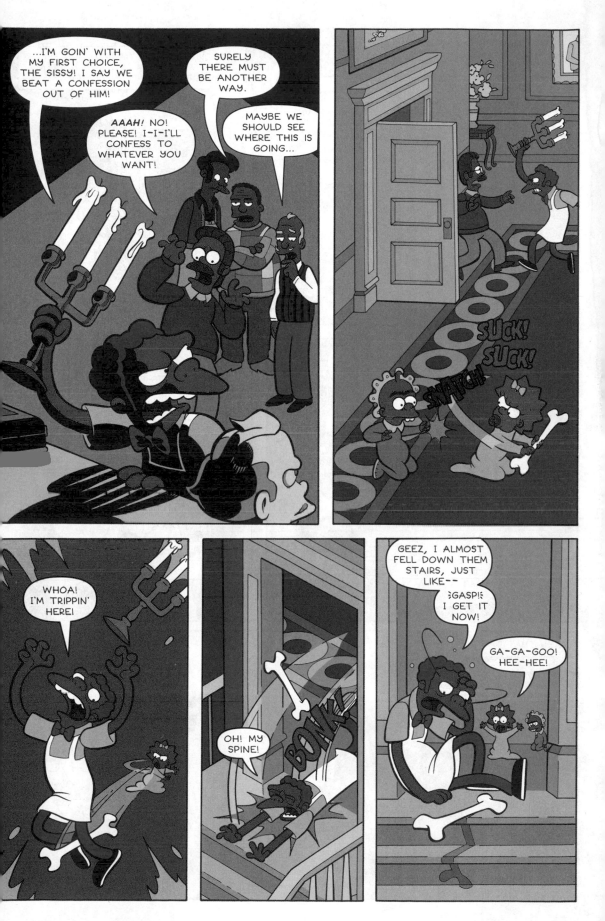

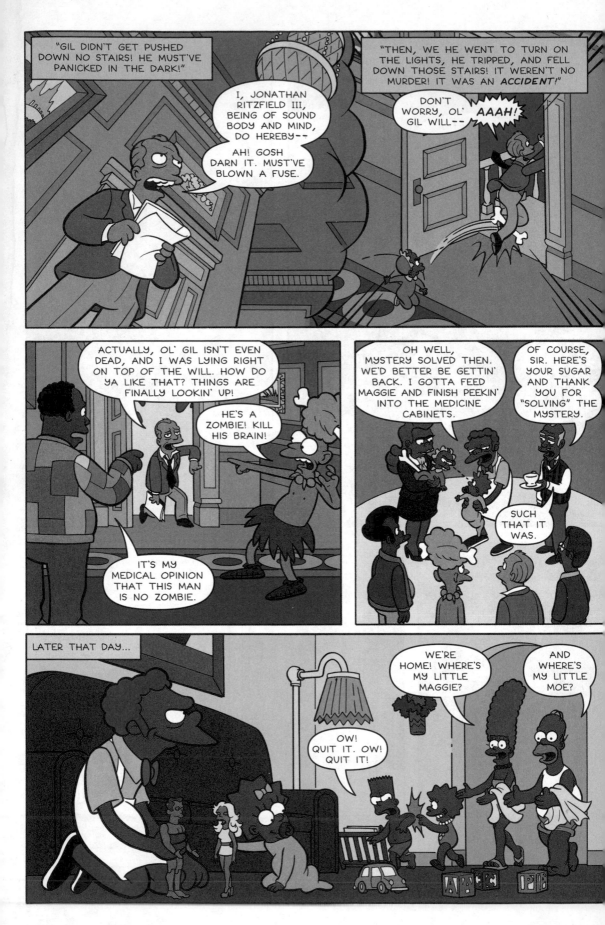

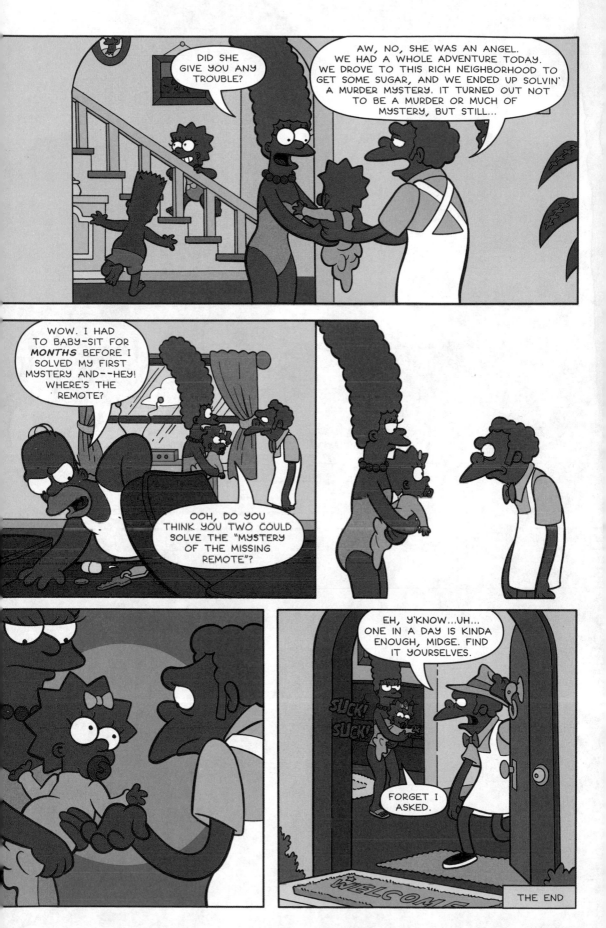

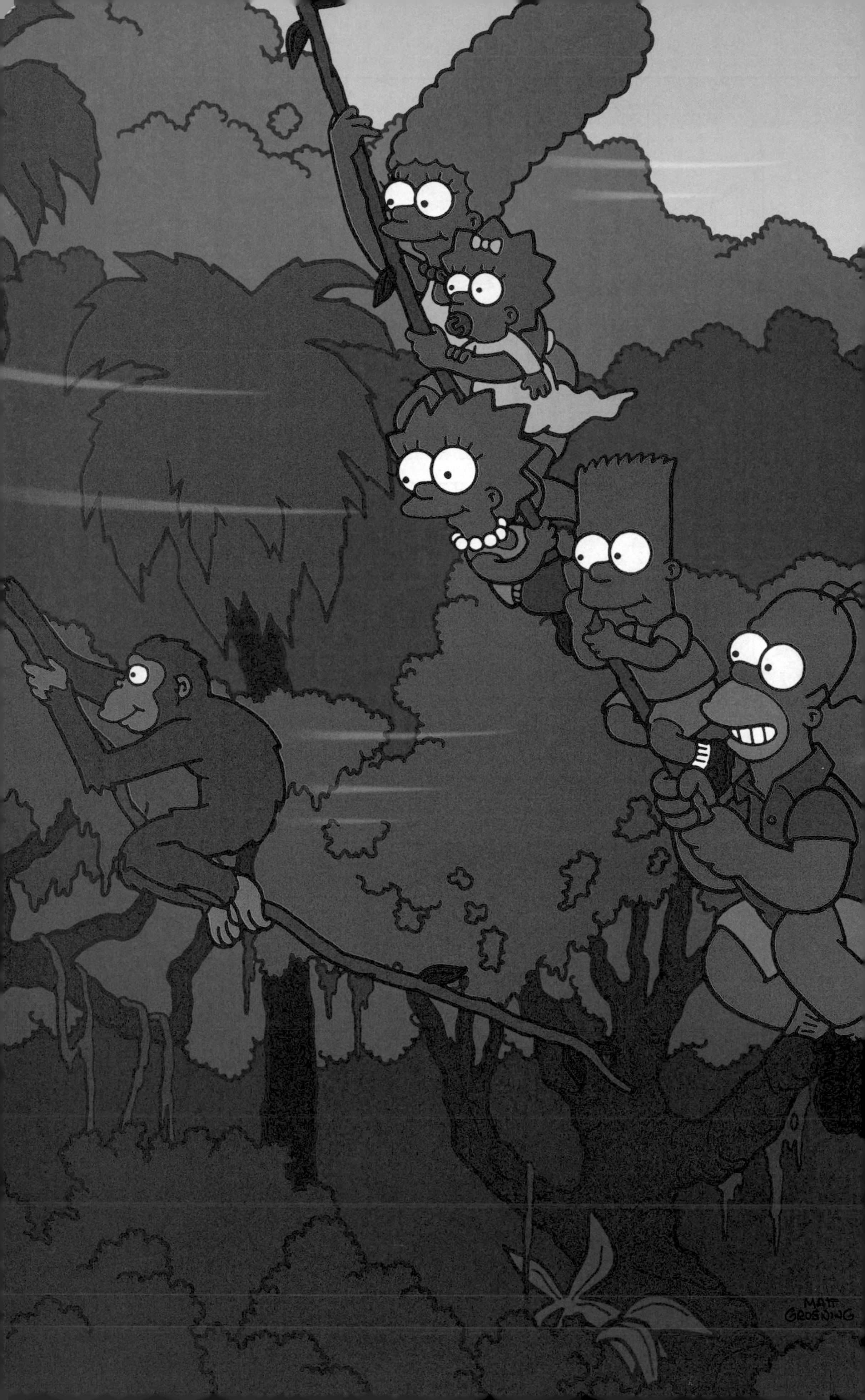
MATT GROENING

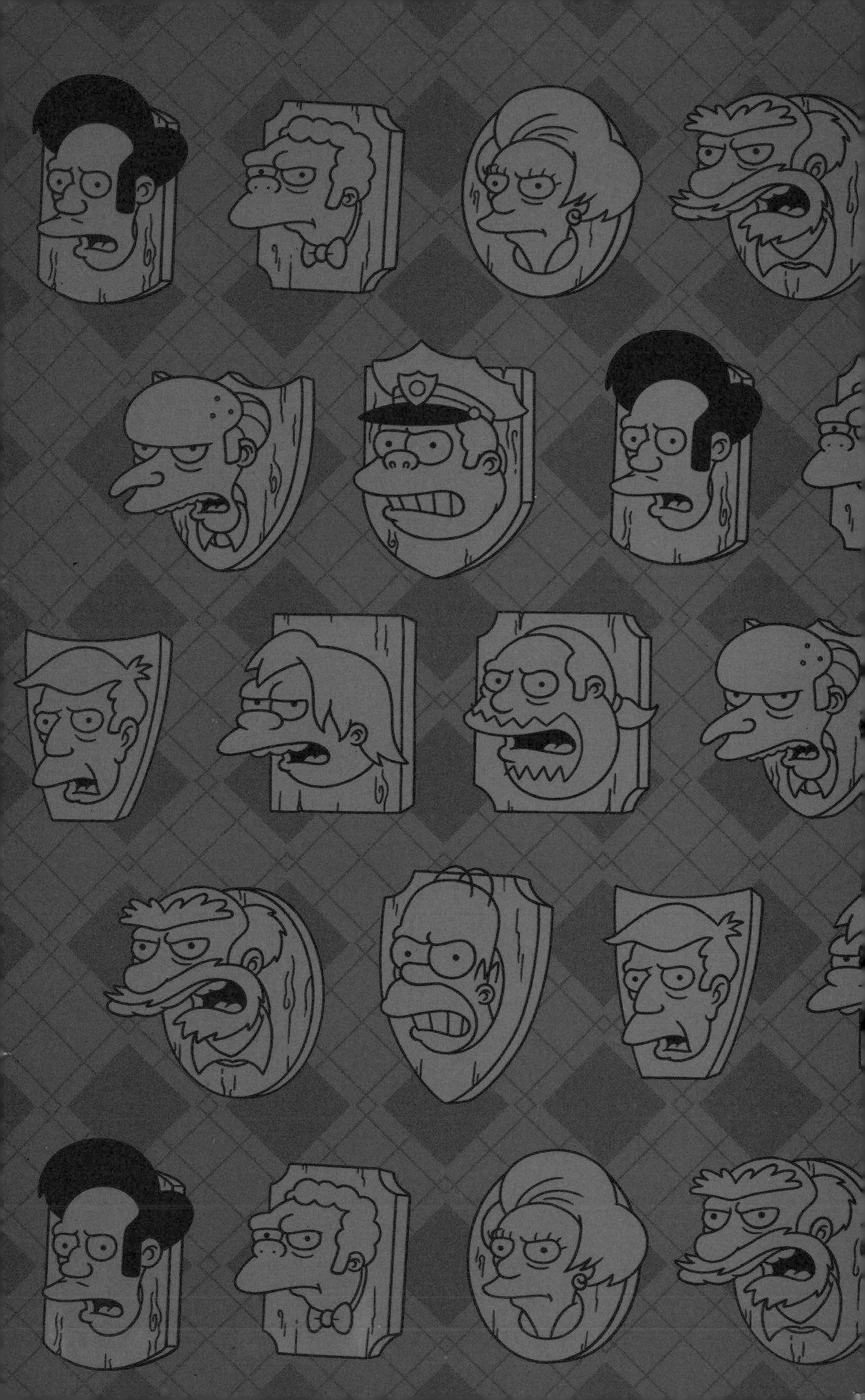